# NURSE NORMA CHRONICLES

## FROM CALL BELLS TO KITCHEN TABLE TALES

BY TAMARA WOODWARD

This is a work of nonfiction. All characters and descriptions of events are the product of the author's imagination and any resemblance to actual persons is entirely coincidental. The information in this book expresses the author's views and opinions and does not necessarily represent the views of any organization.

First published 2025

# DEDICATION

To my Momma B, Sandra Bell (our Sweet Lady):

Your strength is stitched into every chapter of my life. You've been my constant, my compass, and my example of what it means to walk with grace and grit at the same time. This book carries pieces of your wisdom, your laughter, and your prayers between its pages. Thank you for being my forever Sweet Lady.

To my Mother-in-Love, Momma C, Cecelia (our Baby):

You've been our steady rock, pouring out love and support in ways that never go unnoticed. Your presence is proof that family is not only what we're born into, but what we build through love. Thank you for being our Baby, in name and in spirit, always holding us together.

To my Bind, one-legged, allergic-to-everything, best-protector mutt in the world, Kody: Who knew God could send a guardian angel in a furry, sneeze-inducing package? You've been my watchdog, my comic relief, and my furry pillow to cry on. Fierce protector, stubborn sidekick, and four-legged therapist—you've earned your place in these pages more than once.

# TABLE OF CONTENTS

# ACKNOWLEDGMENTS

This book, like every part of my journey, was not built alone.

To my editor — thank you for taking my messy pages and helping me shape them into a story that breathes. You sharpened my words while protecting my voice, and that is a gift I'll never take for granted.

To my family and friends — thank you for cheering me on, even when I was runningon coffee, chaos, and little sleep. Your encouragement kept me standing when I wanted to sit this dream out.

To my Sister-Cousin Shadonne (my Twin) — thank you for being my secret keeper, my motivation, and for always showing up in my life full of love, protection, and grace. You are proof that family is more than blood; it's the bond that carries us through every storm.

To Dr. Brenda (my Dr. B) — you showed me the road map to authorship and guided me with every gentle text and answered phone call until my first book was published. Your wisdom and patience gave me the courage to walk this path, and I am forever grateful.

To my TECU community — you are the heartbeat of this work. Your stories, your laughter, and your resilience remind me every day why I write. You are proof that healing and humor belong in the same room.

Most of all, I thank God for grace — the kind that covers yesterday, strengthens today, and promises brighter tomorrows.

# CHAPTER 1

# THE COVID HALLWAY AND THE MASK REBELLION

I should've known the day was cursed the moment my coffee tasted like Lysol.

Not Lysol exactly—thank the Lord—but the bitter tang of bleach had been clinging to the hospital air since sunrise and somehow seeped right into my cup. That was the thing during the pandemic: everything tasted like antiseptic. Even the vending machine Twinkies tasted like they'd been lovingly wiped down with a Clorox wipe. And gum from my own pocket? Mint with notes of Purell.

Housekeeping had gone from "wipe the counters" to "sanitize like the Pope's coming," and I was grateful... mostly. But after a while, it became impossible to tell where the scent of death ended and the smell of bleach began. Some days, they seemed like the same thing.

"Norma Jean!" My charge nurse hollered from the far end of the unit before my first sip cooled. She had that tone—the one that meant my break, my bladder, and my sanity were already in jeopardy. "You're getting the COVID hallway today!"

Not "the east wing." Not "Hall 4." During the pandemic, we renamed spaces by their level of dread. And the COVID hallway was the kind of assignment you got if you were experienced enough to handle chaos... but not important enough to dodge it.

Walking toward it was like gearing up for battle. The signs along the walls screamed their warnings: ISOLATION --

FULL PPE REQUIRED, REPORT SYMPTOMS

IMMEDIATELY, MINIMIZE CONTACT. Family photos were taped beside some warnings—smiling faces of people who couldn't be there. You'd glance at a baby in a tutu, then hear the patient inside gasping for air, and the air around you would get just a little heavier.

The hallway had a sound to it—an echo of shoe covers on tile, the faint buzz of oxygen machines, and that almost-tooquiet silence right before a monitor started screaming. Every step made the N95 clamp tighter against my cheeks, and every inhale reminded me that this mask was the only thing between me and a virus that had already claimed the lives of coworkers and friends.

Before hitting the door, I ducked into the supply room for gloves and sanitizer. Virgil was already there, wrestling with his isolation gown as if it were a wild animal.

"You know," he said, tugging at the ties, "my father called this morning just to remind me he was performing a highprofile surgery while I'd be... quote... passing out applesauce to contagious patients."

I raised an eyebrow. "And yet here you stand."

Virgil rolled his eyes so hard I thought he'd sprain them. "That man's ego should have its own medical chart. He likes to remind me he was published in The Lancet before he turned thirty. He still signs birthday cards with 'M.D., F.A.C.S., PhD, blah blah blah' like he's worried Hallmark won't recognize his greatness without the credentials."

Lord, have mercy, I thought. If my daddy had bragged like that, my mama would've knocked him upside the head with a cast-iron skillet and told him to take the trash out.

I smirked. "Let me guess—he thinks nursing is beneath you?"

"Beneath him, actually," Virgil said, deadpan. "He once told me—at Thanksgiving, mind you—that Florence Nightingale had more ambition than I do. Then he passed me the cranberry sauce like it was a mic drop."

Florence Nightingale? Really? If anybody tried that in my family, the cranberry sauce would've ended up smeared across the wall. Probably followed by a shoe.

I burst out laughing, nearly dropping the sanitizer. "Did you throw the sauce back at him?"

"Tempting. Instead, I told him I'd rather be the nurse who actually talks to patients than the surgeon who forgets their names after stitching them up. He didn't appreciate that. My mother coughed so hard I thought she was going to need a bronchodilator to cover the silence."

Poor Virgil, I thought. Standing in the shadow of a man who thinks stethoscopes are crowns. No wonder he wrestles gowns like they owe him money.

He gave the gown one final aggressive tug, then shrugged. "So yeah, proving him wrong. Slowly. One applesauce cup at a time."

I strapped on my N95 mask until it bit into my cheekbones, the gloves snapping into place with a crisp little pop. Virgil leaned on his cart, giving me the nurse-to-nurse look. "Here we go." Somewhere down the hall, a man coughed—wet, rattling, and close enough to make both of us shift our stance.

It only took a second to recognize that cough. That gravelly, worn-out wheeze belonged to Reggie, one of the patients I'd met in the ED the week before. Former truck driver, two packs a day for years—the man practically had Marlboro stitched into his lungs. I remembered sitting on the edge of his stretcher while he shook his head and rasped, "Nurse, I've been smoking since Nixon was in office. Two packs a day keep the boredom away—that's what I used to say. Now it feels like I'm hauling eighteen-wheelers on my own chest just trying to breathe."

And yet, I thought, I bet he'd light up tomorrow if somebody offered him one.

Back in the hall, his cough rattled again, echoing off the linoleum like a busted muffler. Lord, here we go again, I thought. Reggie and his two-pack-a-day past just rolled back onto my shift like a bad sequel nobody asked for.

"Norma! Is that you?!" Then coming closer and with a deeper rattle: "Norma Jean Woods!" (My full government name.

Exposed!) "Is that you?!" she hollered.

Afraid to look up, I froze mid-step. Oh no. I knew that voice.

And then I spotted her. Ms. Betty. Of course.

Because God forbid a pandemic put her on mute. She stood in her doorway, hair bonnet half-off, mask not on her face but looped around her neck like a scarf.

Virgil froze. "Oh no. Is this the Ms...?"

Virgil's head tilted. "That's definitely..."

"Ms. Betty," I muttered, and sure enough—there she was.

And at that moment, I knew how my day was going to go.

Then it dawned on me that it was Thursday... It's always a Thursday! The day Satan chases me nonstop for 12 hours straight like I'm the only number in his Rolodex on Thursday. I see you, devil, and not today, Satan. I reject you and all of your attacks. I started praying intensely, as they had instructed us in Bible study, out loud, and repeating 'Holy Spirit Activate' with full and fierce conviction. I said again, 'Holy Spirit, activate!' But I guess today God had decided to check in with someone else because when I opened my eyes...

She stood in her doorway, hair bonnet hanging halfway off, hospital gown untied in the back, and her mask... looped around her neck like a Sunday scarf with a fake cigarette between her fingers that she rolled up from a piece of printer paper.

"Good morning and Happy Thursday, Ms. Betty. Where's your mask?" I asked, trying to keep my voice calm.

She waved it in the air like a victory flag. "Right here! But I ain't wearing it up over my nose—I can't breathe in it. You want me passing out?"

Virgil cleared his throat. "Ma'am, it's hospital policy—"

"Well, sugar, it's my policy to keep my sinuses open. Y'all running around here looking like you're about to rob a bank, and I'm the crazy one?"

Then she did a double take, and her eyes widened as she spotted Virgil correctly and lit up like the Fourth of July.

"Well, hellooo, handsome! Did they finally send me a nurse worth looking at?"

Virgil straightened his gown. "Ma'am, I'm here to help Nurse

Norma today."

She scoffed. "Norma's like family. You? You're new. And fine as wine. Come over here and help me fix this mask before I suffocate."

Her eyes darted to his badge. "Virgil? That's your name? Sounds like you should be driving a tractor, not poking people with needles."

Virgil chuckled politely. "My father's a doctor—" he began.

That was her green light. Her face lit up like she'd just discovered a fresh pot of gossip. She said, "A doctor? Then why are you a nurse?"

Virgil grinned under his mask. "Because I wanted the bedside—the eye contact, the 'you're safe now' approach with my patients. And because I like helping people without charging them a thousand dollars an hour."

Ms. Betty slapped her knee so hard that she hollered loud enough to wake up every patient within a two-room radius. Her IV line jiggled. "Ooooh, child, you just made my day!

I'm telling everybody in this hallway!"

Then, like the diva she was, she straightened her back, smoothed her gown like it was sequined silk, and announced, "By the way, my name ain't no accident. My mama named me after the legendary Betty Boop. Said I came out with big eyes, curly hair, and a scream so high-pitched it could crack a mirror. Baby, I was destined for greatness before I even left the delivery room!"

She fluttered her IV-tethered hand like she was holding a feather boa. "They wanted to name me after my grandma, Mildred. Mildred!" She rolled her eyes so hard her whole head tilted back. "I told my mama later in life, 'Thank you, sugar, for not saddling me with a name that sounds like somebody's Sunday casserole.' Betty got sparkle. Betty got shine. When I walk into a room, people know a legend has arrived!"

Virgil glanced at me with that "do you hear this?" look, but Ms. Betty was already in her own spotlight.

"And don't get it twisted," she added, pointing her two fingers at Virgil like she was blessing him and scolding him all at once. "I may not look like a cartoon, but I am a head-turner. Ask them orderlies—I had three offers of ginger ale just this morning!"

Then she swirled around like a ballerina and yelled to the top of her lungs, lifting one finger in the air: "Room Service

Please and I Thank You, Sir!!"

Lord, give me strength, I thought, biting the inside of my cheek to keep from howling. Only Ms. Betty could turn a hallway into Showtime at the Apollo.

**Coach T says,** *"People think the most challenging part of pandemic nursing was the virus itself. The truth is, some days*

*the real battle was with a stubborn patient and her partially on a mask. But those moments—the belly laughs in between the*

*Chaos—kept us human. In the middle of PPE, policy, and panic, a little humor was the only thing keeping the hallway from swallowing us whole."*

# CHAPTER 2

# THE BED, THE BEEP, AND THE BEAN

I've been floated to the psych ward today, and this is Virgil's regular floor. I'm wondering on the elevator if I'll run into him today. I hate this unit. The first sound that greeted me when the elevator sighed open was a steady, soul-piercing **BEEP—BEEP—BEEP**. If anxiety had a ringtone, this was it.

"Room fourteen," the unit secretary said without glancing up, like a psychic who invoices by the beep. "Been at it since the last ice age."

"I was off for two days," I said. "You telling me it started before I left, and it's still going?"

She slid a cup of pencils toward me like communion. "May the odds be ever in your favor."

I tightened my ponytail, squared my badge, and marched for Room 14 with the grim resolve of a woman already losing three arguments she wasn't present for. The hallway lights hummed. The beeping got louder. Behind me, a visitor whispered, "Is that the fire alarm?" Another answered, "No, that's just healthcare."

Inside 14, the "emergency" looked like this: my patient, **Mr. Slater**, sat upright and cozy, sipping ginger ale with the delicate slurp of a man judging our carbonation choices—rails up. IV pole behaved. Call light untouched. But the bed's exit-alarm box blinked red like I'd caught it doing crimes.

"Morning, Mr. Slater," I sang, reaching for the reset. "How's the—"

"Too sweet," he said, tipping the can. "Y'all changed brands.

This one tastes like you stirred it with a lollipop."

"I'll add 'syrup-forward ginger ale' to today's crises," I said, stabbing reset. The alarm shut up. The room exhaled. I

exhaled. **BEEP—BEEP—BEEP.**

It restarted like it had chased a double espresso.

I traced the sensor-pad cable to the wall, unplugged it, and re-plugged it. Reset. Silence. One Mississippi, two Mississippi—**BEEP.**

"Okay," I said, wearing the polite smile nurses use while negotiating with demons. "We're feisty today."

Mr. Slater pursed his lips. "It's not me. I haven't moved an eyebrow hair for ten minutes."

"You sure?" I lifted the sheet, checking the pad. "The bed thinks you're getting up."

"The bed's wrong," he said. "Also, the bed is rude."

No wrinkles, no crumbs. Reset again. Quiet. Hands on hips. Victory pose. **BEEP—BEEP—BEEP.**

"Sir," I said through teeth, "on a scale from 'STAT' to 'nah,' how committed are you to staying put until PT clears you?"

"Norma," he sighed, "I am a respectable citizen in a backless gown. I'm not training for a 5K."

"Great. Then sit—stay—roll over—good boy."

He snorted. I moved to Step Three in the Ritual of the

Angry

Bed: complete power cycle. Unplug the headboard module. Monitors blink. The room breathed.

I counted to ten, plugged it back in—lights like a Christmas parade. Re-armed the alarm, patted the mattress like a horse.

Silence.

"See?" I whispered to the bed. "We can have nice things."

**BEEP.**

A throat cleared. Virgil leaned in the doorway, gloved hands in pockets, fighting a grin. "I know that sound."

"You also know I'm two beeps away from throwing this bed out the window."

"Don't waste good cardio," he said, rolling in a vitals cart.

"The spirit of the bed is angry. Must be appeased."

"If you brought sage, I'm reporting you to Infection Control."

"No sage. I've got a blood pressure cuff and a whale-song playlist. We'll coax it into peace."

Mr. Slater eyed us. "If you're performing an exorcism, do I get a say?"

"You get front-row seats," I said. "You caused this by existing."

Virgil checked the vitals while I re-ran the checklist: the cords were snug, the pad was centered, and the threshold was correct. I even swapped the sensor cable.

Silence. Precious, blessed silence.

We held our breath. **BEEP.**

"Okay," Virgil said gently, the tone used for toddlers about to lick sockets, "what if it's not the bed?"

I eyed the blinking LED. "What would it be—lighting?

Weather? Mercury in retrograde?"

"User error," Mr. Slater offered, sipping soda like a talkshow host.

Virgil crouched. "Sometimes the pad reads pressure changes from—" He paused. Tilted his head. "Huh."

"What 'huh'?"

He lifted the sheet at the foot of the bed, flashlight ready.

Froze. "Norma, don't overreact."

"I am a professional," I said. *I only scream during my break.*

Something shifted near Mr. Slater's calves—a bundled, warm loaf resettling in an oven. The bed chimed again:

**BEEP—BEEP—BEEP**.

"Sir," I said slowly, eyes on the lump, "are you... alone?"

Mr. Slater went innocent in the way only the guilty can.

"Alone? Like... spiritually?"

"Like physically."

A tiny, indignant sneeze peeped from under the sheet.

I closed my eyes. "Sir. Is there... a living, breathing, bingosized creature in this bed with you?"

Silence. Then a busted sigh. "He's quiet. Mostly."

Virgil's eyes widened. "Oh, you did not."

A cinnamon-colored head the size of a fist popped out, eyes glossy and bold, sweater pink and undeniable.

"Is that a dog?" I asked in the same pitch we use when discovering deli sandwiches in a bedside table.

"He's my emotional support angel," Mr. Slater said. "His name is **Bean**."

Bean blinked, yawned, and—outraged by our disrespect for his contributions to modern medicine—gave the alarm his

tiniest growl. **BEEP—BEEP—BEEP.**

Virgil first bit to stop laughing. I didn't bother. I sat in the visitor chair and let my forehead fall into my palm.

"Mr. Slater, this is a hospital, not a pet motel."

"He's family."

"He's a chihuahua."

"Exactly."

Virgil turned to "check cords" and whispered, "I love Bean personally. Professionally, I did not see Bean."

"Professionally," I said louder, "we're following policy.

Bean goes to a chair at the nurse's station until your daughter comes."

"He'll be frightened," Mr. Slater protested.

"So am I," Virgil said, hand to chest.

Bean squinted at me like I was at best an intern. I scooped him anyway. He weighed approximately two whispers and a secret. Bones printed on the sweater; tag read **BEAN — I'M SMALL BUT I'M LOUD.** *Accurate.*

"Five minutes," I said. "We'll keep him warm and famous. Call your daughter."

Virgil snugged the sensor pad and re-armed the alarm while I tucked Bean into my jacket like a marsupial. The bed fell silent—as if we'd removed the poltergeist. *Imagine that.*

We turned to go just as Maintenance stormed in, like a twoperson SWAT team: tool belts, safety glasses, the swagger of people who hadn't been living with the beep for an hour.

"You called a bed alarm?" the tall one asked.

"Past tense," Virgil said. "We **had** a bed alarm." "We solved it," I added.

He looked wounded. "We solve things for a living."

"Fair," I said. "This one turned out to be... a weightdistribution anomaly."

"Like a bad pad?" the short one squinted.

"Like eight pounds of opinion in a sweater," Virgil said.

They stared at Bean. Bean stared back like he signed their checks.

"We'll document that as 'foreign object interference,'" the tall one said.

"Please do not write 'Bean was foreign to the bed,'" I replied. They left. We left. Bean sneezed.

At the desk, the secretary clocked the lump in the jacket and sighed. "Not again."

"How many Beans have we had?" I asked.

"Three Beans, two Cupcakes, one Sir Lancelot, and a guinea pig named Debra," she said. "Debra was fast. Debra was angry."

We lined a spare tub with a blanket; Bean perched on the rim like a monarch on a balcony. A visitor whispered,

"Therapy dog?"

"No," I said. "Unlicensed consultant."

The visitor took a picture anyway. Bean posed.

Mr. Slater's daughter arrived ten minutes later with a tiny carrier printed with cartoon tacos. "I'm so sorry—Dad asked me to hold Bean while he checked in. He... talked me into it."

"Bean or your father?" I asked.

"Yes," she said.

Bean rode off in his taco Uber with a farewell treat (sue me).

I returned to 14 to find the alarm light a docile green; Mr.

Slater looked both relieved and a touch bereft.

"You okay?" I checked his IV.

He lifted a shoulder. "Hospital feels louder without him."

"It's objectively quieter."

"That's what I mean."

I softened. "We'll get you a new ginger ale. Less lollipop."

He nodded—grateful, a little embarrassed—the way people look when their coping mechanism just toddled out in a sweater.

**Coach T says,** *"Some alarms mean danger. Some mean 'look closer.' The beeping bed wasn't about hardware—it was about a man who needed comfort and a tiny dog who supplied it. In a world of constant noise, notice what quiets you. Keep the policy, yes—but keep the humanity, too."*

# CHAPTER 3

# THE SHORT STRAW SHIFT

If you've never worked a hospital morning shift after a night of chaos, you might think it starts with something noble—a nurse making rounds, a doctor checking vitals, a quiet hum of professionalism.

No.

It starts with coffee.

Coffee is the currency of survival. Coffee is the IV drip for your soul. Coffee is the only reason half the staff hasn't been arrested for assault before 9 a.m.

On that particular morning, the line for the coffee cart wrapped around like it was a jazz concert. The smell of overworked espresso machines mixed with the faint tang of hand sanitizer and the low murmur of caffeine desperation filled the air.

Word had gotten out—like a full-blown hospital plague—that the cart had **complimentary flavored creamer pods.** Hazelnut, vanilla, even that seasonal pumpkin spice that people treat like contraband. It was strictly first-come, first-served, and once they were gone, you were left with sad, plain half-and-half and broken dreams.

Staff were stuffing pods into their pockets, badge lanyards, and God knows where else. I watched one resident slide two French vanilla straight into the side of his scrub pants, as if he were smuggling diamonds. Another nurse cradled a handful like communion wafers.

Meanwhile, the cafeteria cleaning lady—our unofficial security guard—was circling with her spray bottle and rag, wiping the counter as if she were polishing the crown jewels, side-eyeing anyone who reached for "just one more." Every time she caught a hand sneaking back for seconds, she snapped, "One per cup, baby. One."

But the thieves were relentless. A tech shoved three hazelnuts into her bra, as if she were planning for winter. Somebody's intern whispered, "Meet me later, I got a mocha." The black market for creamer was thriving.

And the worst part? We all had to be in the **assignment huddle** in minutes. Which meant the race was on: either you grabbed your caffeine fix now or you walked into the huddle raw, creamerless, and already mad at the world.

By the time my turn at the cart finally came, the clock was already mocking me. Huddle in five minutes. Coffee line at a standstill. Flavored creamer pods are dwindling like the last lifeboats on the Titanic.

I snatched a vanilla pod, slammed it into my cup like a shot of salvation, and took off down the hall. Around me, staff was hustling toward the huddle, balancing cups in one hand and clipboards in the other, trying not to baptize their scrubs in scalding espresso.

It looked like a caffeinated relay race. One nurse powerwalked with her coffee held aloft like the Olympic torch. A respiratory therapist stuffed three creamers into his shoe mid-stride. Somebody's cup lid popped, and hazelnut foam splattered the wall—a casualty of war.

We barreled toward the huddle room, caffeine sloshing, masks slipping, badge lanyards swinging like medals we didn't want. The only rule was simple: don't be late, don't spill on your scrubs, and for the love of God, don't lose your one free pod before the charge nurse starts passing out doom.

Every morning, like soldiers lining up for battle, the oncoming crew gathers in a crooked circle around the charge nurse. Clipboards clutched. Pens ready. Eyes glazed. The night shift rattles off reports like an auctioneer, and the rest of us pray for mercy.

Princess Neuongu, my lovely Nigerian nurse sister, slid in beside me, her mask askew, her curls pulled into a bun that already screamed, "Don't test me." She nudged my elbow with her cup. "If we don't end up on the same unit today, I'm faking chest pain."

"Make it convincing," I muttered, sipping my vanilla lifeline. "They'll probably give you a bed alarm."

Our charge nurse cleared her throat, her mask puffing out with the force of someone who already hated today. "We're short again. Three call-outs. ICU is pulling one of ours for a sitter, and there's a double admit coming up."

A collective groan rolled through the group like a wave.

Assignments were passed out like sentencing. "Room 2

through 6, you've got post-op." "Room 7 through 10, you've got med-surg overflow. Lovely, you're with orthopedics today." Then her eyes slid to me.

"Norma Jean, you're on the COVID hallway."

Again.

Lovely hissed into her mask. "Orthopedics? Knees and hips?

Girl, I didn't stretch this morning!" I squeezed her arm.

"Better than the alternative."

The unit exhaled like they'd just dodged a bullet. I swore I heard someone whisper, "Thank you, Jesus."

The charge nurse looked down again. "Norma Jean Woods—

I said you're on the COVID hallway."

Yes ma'am. I sank into my chair. "Always on a Thursday," I muttered.

I pasted on a brave little nod; the kind nurses do when our soul is saying, *Why me, Lord?* It was Thursday, which made perfect sense. Thursdays were when Satan flipped through his

Rolodex and found my name highlighted in neon.

"Mask up, gown up, glove up," the charge nurse barked.

"And stay safe."

Stay safe. Translation: *You're on your own, sweetheart.*

And with that, we scattered—half to charts, half to chaos, and me straight to the one thing standing between me and the abyss: more coffee.

The COVID hallway was its own level of the underworld. Not "Hall 4" or "East Wing"—we named areas by their dread. level, and this one was the boss fight. It was where assignments went when your experience was high enough to handle chaos, but your political clout was too low to dodge it.

Lovely walked with me as far as the split in the hallway, both of us juggling cold coffee and fresh dread. She bumped her shoulder into mine. "If we don't make it out of here, tell my mama I went down fighting."

I smirked under my N95. "Girl, you're going to ortho. You'll be buried in hips and knees. I'm the one heading into Dante's Inferno."

She groaned, dramatically clutching her chest. "And that's exactly why I wanted us on the same unit. We could've tagteamed Satan."

We reached the fork—she veered toward ortho, I turned toward isolation. "Love you, sis," she called over her shoulder.

"Love you back," I said. "Don't sprain your back lifting hips."

Walking toward the COVID zone felt like marching into a war movie. **ISOLATION** signs screamed from the doors.

The air was heavy—not just with sickness, but with fear.

PPE crinkled with every step. Somewhere behind a closed door, a monitor beeped in erratic bursts, the rhythm already in my bones.

My face shield fogged instantly as the first door closed behind me. The hiss of oxygen, the muffled coughs, the plastic rustle of gowns brushing past—all of it blurred into the soundtrack of this hallway.

It hit just as I was mentally mapping my patient list: Code

**Blue, room 412.**

Everything shifted. The hallway transformed into a perfectly choreographed ballet of urgency: PPE snapping into place, gurneys rattling, the crash cart slamming against the wall as if it knew its mark. Someone shouted for EPI, someone else was already pushing chest compressions, and I found my place in the dance without thinking.

The call crackled overhead—**"Code Blue, Room 412."**

I dropped my coffee on the nurse's station, the splash forgotten before it even hit the floor, and sprinted down the hall. By the time I pushed through the door, the room had already transformed into a stage—every player stepping into their role with practiced precision.

The patient: a **22-year-old female**, chest rising in shallow spasms before collapsing into stillness. Too young. Far too young.

The respiratory therapist was already at the head of the bed, mask sealed, bag-valve pumping in a steady rhythm, each squeeze timed like a percussion beat. "I've got the airway," he called, his voice calm but urgent.

A nurse pressed hard and fast into compressions, arms locked, body moving like a piston. The bed rattled beneath the force, the monitor shrieking in counterpoint.

"Epi ready," another nurse announced, syringe poised, waiting for the doctor's cue.

The doctor's voice cut clear, the conductor of this impossible ballet. "Two milligrams IV push. Continue compressions.

Don't stop."

And we didn't, not for a heartbeat.

I took my place at the side, sliding into the choreography without thought. Hands moved, gloves snapped, IV ports flushed. The crash cart drawers slammed open and shut with the rhythm of cymbals. Pads slapped against bare skin. "Charging to 200. Clear!" The body jolted, then settled, the air thick with burnt ozone and sweat.

Every movement was sharp, synchronized—the kind of seamless teamwork that only appears when lives hang in the balance. No hesitation. No wasted breath. Just muscle memory honed from too many nights like this, too many bodies on too many beds.

It was, in its way, **a ballet**—not graceful, but relentless—a choreography born of desperation and training, equal parts science and instinct. The RT nods to me to switch places. The quiet handoff of the ambu bag. The firm squeeze of my shoulder from a colleague who said, You've *got the next round, I've got you covered.*

Minutes stretched into lifetimes. Sweat dripped down brows under fogging shields. The monitor screamed, then stuttered, then teased us with a rhythm.

"Pulse check," the doctor snapped.

Fingers pressed to a carotid. A beat. Then another. A fragile, miraculous flutter under the skin.

"She's back," someone breathed, the words heavy with relief and exhaustion.

The room exhaled all at once—the way an audience does when the curtain finally falls.

I stepped back, chest heaving, gloves trembling, and caught the eyes of my coworkers above their masks. Nothing needed to be said. We knew. We had done what we could, and for now—for this moment—it was enough.

By the time I staggered back to the nurse's station, my coffee was ice cold, my hair plastered to my forehead, and my pulse still trying to catch up. Lovely appeared a few minutes later, mask hanging off one ear, eyes wide over the rim of her cup.

"Girl, you okay?" she said, voice low but steady. "We heard it from ortho. Code Blue Covid Isolation Unit. Y'all sounded like a NASCAR pit crew on fire. I ran over to see if you made it out. For what it's worth, Norma Jean Woods, you're amazing if no one ever tells you, sis, remember I just did."

I dropped into the nearest chair I saw and said, 'Thank you, sis.' And yes, the drama follows me on this unit like a stigma. "But at least the choreography was tight."

Lovely gave me a tired and proud grin with the "YOU GOT THIS, SIS" side eye and nudged my cold cup toward me. "It's cold, but drink it anyway. We've still got a whole act left in this circus."

After the adrenaline of the Code Blue drained out of my veins, I leaned against the wall outside the room, catching my breath. The unit was already buzzing again—monitors chirping, call lights pinging—like nothing monumental had just happened. That's the cruelty of hospital life: the world doesn't pause, even when you've just dragged someone back from the edge.

That's when Kayla—one of our newer nurses, her eyes still too wide, too hopeful—sidled up next to me. Her gloves were trembling just enough that she tried to hide her hands in her pockets.

"Norma," she whispered, voice low so it wouldn't crack, "do you ever... You know... get scared you're not enough?"

I knew what she meant. Not *enough skill.* She was sharp; her hands had been steady during compressions. What she meant was *enough to survive this job and still be a whole person at the end of the day.*

I didn't answer right away. Instead, I tipped my head toward the supply closet. We slipped inside, shutting the door on the chaos. The air smelled like alcohol wipes and cardboard. We perched on overturned glove boxes like kids hiding from chores.

"Kayla," I said, my voice softer now, "the trick isn't to get scared. Fear is baked into this job. The trick is showing

up anyway—even when your hands shake, even when your chest feels hollow, even when you've cried yourself hoarse in the car before walking inside."

Her chin trembled. She blinked fast, fighting it—then the tears broke free. She pressed her mask against her cheeks as if it could hold her together, but it couldn't.

I reached over and squeezed her shoulder. "And listen—when you can't show up anymore, you don't quit. You ask for help. From your team. From me. You don't carry this alone."

Her breath hitched, then steadied—two nurses in a tiny closet, mascara running like we'd been dumped on prom night. No words for a while, just shared silence and the rhythm of our breathing.

And somehow, in that cramped little space, something stitched itself back together—not just for her, but for me too.

I saw it in her eyes when she finally looked up: Kayla wasn't going to break today. She was going to bend, wobble maybe, but not break.

And in that moment, I knew—she'd be mine to mentor. My protégé. The one I'd teach the ropes to, the one I'd show how to fight the darkness without letting it swallow you whole.

The Code Blue had given her her first scar. Now it was my job to help her turn it into armor.

**Coach T says***: In nursing, people think the most challenging part is facing the blood, the sweat, the endless alarms. But the truth? It's moments like this—standing shoulder to shoulder with your team, fighting to bring a 22-year-old back when her life is hanging by a thread. That's when you realize this work is not random chaos. It's a dance. Every nod, every squeeze, every push of a syringe—it's choreography with life itself.*

*And when the pulse returns, even faint, even fragile, you don't just feel relief. You feel the weight of what it means to be human together. These moments don't leave us when the shift ends. We carry them home, in our bones and in our prayers. Because the truth is—in that room, under those lights—none of us danced alone.*

# CHAPTER 4

# WHEN THE SHIFT HITS THE FAN

The shift hit the fan at exactly 7:12 a.m.

I know because I had just taken my first blessed sip of coffee—the kind that's hot enough to burn your esophagus but still worth it—when the overhead speakers crackled like Satan himself was trying to clear his throat. Static coughed through the hospital, followed by a muffled voice:

"Uh... Attention staff... never mind."

And then they forgot to let go of the mic. For three whole seconds, the entire hospital got treated to the sound of somebody's labored, wheezy breathing.

"Off to a great start," I muttered into my cup.

Of course, I was on assignment in the ED that day—the Emergency Department, where chaos is the house wine and nobody ever drinks just one glass. You don't walk into the ED so much as surrender to it. Forget easing into your shift. The second you badge in, it's like getting dropped into the spin cycle of a washing machine.

Sure enough, I wasn't even on the clock five minutes when the triage doors swung open and dumped an entire wedding party into the waiting room like we were hosting some halfprice Vegas chapel special.

The bride was still in a silk robe, mascara streaks running like battle paint. Two bridesmaids were sobbing into each other's arms. And the groom? Poor thing was clutching his own bouquet like it was a flotation device and he was already drowning.

"What happened?" I asked, already bracing myself.

"The mother of the bride," the groom stammered. "She... she fainted."

Before I could even react, the mother herself stormed into view, rhinestones flashing, hairspray shellacked, and indignation at full throttle. "I did not faint," she announced to the entire waiting room. "I swooned. There's a difference."

She slapped a hand dramatically to her chest. "Also, I can't breathe—my left arm tingles. My head feels like I'm trapped inside a marching band. And someone stole my purse."

The bride burst into fresh sobs. The mother waved her off as if she were a mosquito. "Save it for the aisle, Tiffany." Then she looked straight at me. "Nurse, I'll need an IV, three of your strongest nurses, and a fan."

"It's February," I said flatly.

"Then a brochure," she snapped. "I can fan myself."

Meanwhile, the rest of the waiting room was already a carnival of questionable life choices. A man sat with a fishhook dangling from his ear like DIY jewelry. ("Don't ask," he muttered, which of course made me want to.) A preschooler perched on his mother's lap while she whispered, "He swallowed a marble, but it's a small marble."

And in the corner, a teenage boy held his obviously broken wrist and kept repeating, "It's not broken," like denial was an acceptable splint.

And here's the kicker: all of this? The fainting, the swooning, the missing purse, the marble kid, the broken-wrist boy? This was just the waiting room.

I tightened my ponytail, took another gulp of lava coffee, and headed to the nurse's station to grab my assignments, already knowing today was going to chew me up and spit me out.

Naturally, the printer decided to die on impact.

It coughed, spat out half a page, and froze. The screen flashed a message that Dante himself could've written:

ERROR 41: PAPER JAM IN THE FOURTH CIRCLE OF HELL.

"Relatable," I muttered.

I yanked the tray, fished out tiny paper confetti, and whispered a desperate prayer. The printer ignored me with the cold indifference of every machine that knows it owns your soul.

And that was all before 7:20 a.m.

Behind me, chaos had already started brewing like a bad pot of decaf. A family had formed a semicircle around the triage nurse, holding a smartphone up like it were the holy text. On the screen, glowing bright blue, was the unmistakable font of WebMD doom.

"My uncle has all of these," the self-appointed family spokesman declared, scrolling aggressively, "which means he has this."

The triage nurse blinked, halfway between polite and homicidal. "He... has anxiety."

"Exactly," the nephew said, jabbing the screen. "And according to this, anxiety can be fatal if left un-Googled."

"Untreated," I corrected gently.

He nodded, like we were colleagues. "Right, untreated. So, we need the tests that prove it's not the fatal kind."

I pinched the bridge of my nose. "What fatal kind?"

He scrolled again, eyes darting like he was searching for a lottery number. "Here—look. It's right between 'stress' and 'numb toes.'" He turned the screen toward me, triumphant.

"Acute catastrophic heart brain."

I stared at the words. "That's... not a thing."

"It's on the internet," he shot back, with the confidence of a man holding a receipt from God.

"Exactly," I said, and smiled the kind of smile that said I had chosen peace even if it killed me.

Meanwhile, the waiting room orchestra played on. At 7:29, a stretcher rolled by with an elderly man whose granddaughter had looped his oxygen tubing into a bow—because nothing says 'stability' like accessory flair. At 7:34, the call-light board lit up like a Vegas slot machine. At 7:38, the brand-new interpreter iPad refused to connect to Wi-Fi because, apparently, it "couldn't detect the concept of the internet."

So there I was, standing in a waiting room that looked more like a live-action soap opera, dealing with a bride's mother who demanded both an IV and a fan brochure, a fishhook patient sulking like Captain Ahab's understudy, a marble- swallowing preschooler grinning like this was recess, a broken-wrist teenager in complete denial, and now, WebMD Nephew, who had diagnosed his uncle with a disease that sounded like Dr. Seuss wrote it.

All before 8:00 a.m.

I gripped my lukewarm coffee, squared my shoulders, and muttered the same mantra I always did in the ED: choose chaos, but make it look professional.

At 7:41 on the dot, the door to the supply cabinet slammed open like it owed somebody rent. Malik, our respiratory therapist with the patience of a saint and the temper of a storm cloud, came barreling in.

"Where are the good neb masks?" he hissed, eyes wild.

"Don't tell me we're out."

The cabinet stared back at him, empty as a politician's promise.

"I ordered them," I said, holding up both hands like I was innocent.

"So did I," Malik snapped. "Three times. Apparently, the supply chain is now a rumor."

He rubbed his temples with the kind of long-suffering sigh

that sounded like it was pulled from the Book of Job. Malik had been here long enough to grow a second spine, and today it was bending.

"Okay," I said, trying to sound optimistic. "We can pivot."

He leveled me with a look. "Norma, I pivoted so much yesterday my hips are filing a grievance."

I laughed. He didn't.

We compromised with a stash of pediatric neb masks—the tiny ones shaped like dragons that hissed when you turned them on. Not ideal for grown men with COPD, but desperate times call for desperate reptiles.

Malik held one up, the plastic dragon head glaring in his palm. "May the baby dragon gods have mercy."

He stalked off, muttering like he was about to summon a séance.

I leaned against the counter, watching him disappear into the chaos, and thought: This is the ED in one scene. We're out of the basics, but we'll MacGyver it with cartoon equipment and a touch of sarcasm. And somehow, it'll still work.

By 8:06, though, even sarcasm couldn't keep pace. The shift officially went haywire.

I had just settled at the desk to bang out a chart note when a nurse's shout ricocheted down the corridor: "Watch your step!"

Too late.

A tray of half-melted ice had exploded across the linoleum like it was auditioning for the Winter Olympics. Cubes scattered in every direction, spreading faster than gossip at a family reunion.

A volunteer lunged with a mop and immediately turned the place into a slip-'n'-slide. A phlebotomist tried to dodge the puddle and ended up moonwalking unintentionally, arms flailing like he was channeling Michael Jackson. A visitor in flip-flops shrieked and latched onto a vending machine like it was her last dance partner on Earth.

And because this was the ER, where logic comes to die, someone had parked a housekeeping cart directly in front of the only working blood pressure machine. Taped to the handle was a sticky note in loopy handwriting: OUT OF ORDER BECAUSE SHE'S TIRED.

I blinked at it, muttering, "Same, ma'am. Same."

Before I could even finish the thought, the overhead speakers coughed back to life.

"Code S—" they sputtered, then cut out.

Half the hallway froze.

"Code what?" someone whispered.

"Sandwich?" a tech guessed hopefully. "Because I could go for."

The mic screeched back on, loud enough to rattle fillings:

"CODE STROKE, ROOM 18. CODE STROKE, ROOM 18."

And just like that, the circus turned into a sprint.

Malik shot past me, neb cart rattling behind him like a battle chariot. The charge nurse was already barking orders into the phone. The CT tech materialized at the doorway like a relay runner waiting for the handoff.

We piled into Room 18—me, Malik, two nurses, and a doctor whose coffee was still steaming in his hand.

The patient—a man in his sixties—stared blankly at the

ceiling, half his face slack, the other half fighting to hold on. His wife clutched the bedrail, lips moving in prayer, eyes wide enough to hold every fear she'd ever carried.

The rhythm of a Code Stroke isn't dramatic—it's drilled. FAST: Face, Arms, Speech, Time. Call. Assess. Move. And pray the doors cooperate.

They did.

We had him on a stretcher and flying toward CT in seconds. Monitors beeped, gown flapped like a flag of surrender, wheels shrieked against tile.

His wife stumbled after us, voice cracking. "Is this my fault?"

I slowed just long enough to look her in the eye. "No. This is your husband's brain asking for help. We're answering."

Her chin trembled. "Even if he yelled at you?" "Especially then," I said.

And then we were gone—swallowed by the rush of wheels, the crackle of radios, and the kind of urgency that steals the air right out of your chest.

This day had already ambushed me. No easing into the shift, no gentle warm-up. Just me, walking in with a lukewarm coffee, trying to convince myself this was the day I'd pace my steps, sip water, and maybe avoid getting yelled at by anyone over 80. Spoiler: all three goals would be missed by noon.

The rest of the shift tried to outdo itself in absurdity, but then... I got assigned to Mr. Lewis. He was in his 70s, softspoken, the kind of patient who apologized every time you came in the room. He was recovering from pneumonia and just needed monitoring.

"Thanks for being here," he said quietly as I adjusted his oxygen.

"That's my job," I replied.

"No," he said, shaking his head. "You've got... I don't know... a kindness. And in a place like this, that's rare."

It stopped me cold. After a day of being screamed at, tripped over, and pulled into dramas I didn't start, here was someone seeing me not as the uniform, not as the role, but as a human being who gave a damn.

I smiled, adjusted his blanket, and felt my feet root back into the floor. This was why I stayed.

**Coach T Says:** *When the shift hits the fan, remember: the drama will end, the mess will get cleaned, and someone, somewhere, will be grateful you showed up. Hang on for that moment—it's the gold buried in the garbage.*

# CHAPTER 5

# CHAOS, CUPCAKES & COMPASSION

The day didn't even wait for patients to start acting up—the staff clock beat them to it.

At exactly 6:58 a.m., the hallway outside the ED looked like a Black Friday line at Walmart. Nurses, techs, and respiratory staff were stacked shoulder to shoulder, each clutching their badge like it was a golden ticket. Everyone wanted the same thing: to clock in before the system docked them for being late.

But the time-punch machine? Oh, she had other plans.

The little screen blinked an error message in that smug corporate font: SYSTEM UNAVAILABLE. PLEASE TRY AGAIN LATER.

"Later?" Sharon barked, already ten decibels too high for this hour. "I'm here NOW. Later doesn't pay my rent!"

A chorus of groans rose. Someone slapped the side of the machine as if it were a stubborn vending machine. Another nurse held her badge to the reader so long that the plastic started to warp from the heat of her frustration.

Meanwhile, Malik leaned against the wall, arms folded, sipping his coffee like this was better than Netflix. "Y'all realize HR is gonna say this is our fault somehow, right?"

"HR can kiss my—" Sharon started, but the machine beeped. Everyone froze.

For one glorious second, it looked like it had accepted a badge. Then it spat out a slip of paper that read: ERROR 666:

DEVICE POSSESSED. CONTACT EXORCIST.

The hallway went wild. People were swearing in three different languages, waving badges in the air like a protest march. Somebody yelled, "We need a priest!" and I swear half of them meant it.

I just stood there with my coffee, watching the circus unfold, and thought: This is how you know it's gonna be one of those shifts.

The ED doors whooshed open, as if they were tired of keeping secrets. I was two sips into a coffee that tasted like a grudge when the morning decided to become daytime television.

Sequins hit first.

Two men in full sparkle strutted in like the runway had potholes. One wore a bright fuchsia feather boa that molted like stressed-out parrots; the other had a rhinestone sash that read QUEEN OF THE EASTERN SHORE in letters big enough to file an insurance claim against.

"Marco," said the first man, adjusting his feathered accessory, "I told you not to speak to me until I've had peanuts or absolution."

"Then confess, Lenny," Marco snapped, "because the vending machine takes cash, not apologies."

Behind them, a white man with a day-old shave and a toddler on his hip did the panicked parent sway, the one that says Please, someone older than me, take charge. A Black grandma in a white church hat drifted behind in their wake, whispering scripture like the room owed her tithes.

Security muttered, "Norma, if you're gonna run, now's the cardio window."

"Sweetie, I am the cardio window," I said, slapping on a smile and my triage badge. "Let's breathe, people. One at a time, or I'm issuing numbers like the deli."

Lenny spun, feathers floating, voice vibrating glass. "We would be calm, nurse, if a certain alleged caretaker hadn't abandoned my god-niece for karaoke night."

"Alleged?!" Marco clutched imaginary pearls. "Miss Delilah was present. I left a note."

A beat. From the automatic doors came the sharp click of determined heels on linoleum. Enter Miss Delilah: tall, gorgeously padded, curls like a choir, lashes with their own weather system. She wore a denim jacket with patches that said things like "FRAGILE BUT FABULOUS" and "HANDLE WITH CARE OR ELSE."

She flung a glittery tote onto a chair. "The note said—and I quote—'Be right back, BRB, promise.' I Googled your promise, and it returned three hours and fifty-two minutes."

The toddler—little girl, pinafore, curls that didn't care about anyone's drama—hid her face in her blanket and peeped at me with saucer eyes.

I crouched. "Hey, cupcake. I'm Norma. You like juice? I have the good kind—apple that's half juice, half sugar, and a prayer."

She nodded. I slid her a box, the staff-fridge contraband. She sipped like it held peace.

"Vitals here," I said to the adults, already cuffing grandma's arm. "Who has chest pain? Who has hurt feelings? They are not billed the same."

"I have betrayal," Miss Delilah announced, hand to clavicle. "And a blister. These heels were meant for a twenty-minute exit, not a hostage situation."

"Betrayal's out-of-network," I said. "Blister, I can do."

Behind me, the waiting room's drama was warming up. An interracial couple at two o'clock—a Black woman in scrubs, a white man in a landscaping tee—were arguing in whispershouts.

"I texted you twice," she said, jaw set. "My mother sat with the baby for three hours."

"I was stuck in traffic," he said, palms up.

"On your couch?"

"It was emotional traffic."

I sighed. "Y'all, I don't have a form for emotional traffic. But I can offer a chair, a water, and an 'inside voices' sticker if you earn it."

They blinked, chastened, and took their seats. I handed over two paper cups, as if I were baptizing them.

"Back to the script," I told the sequin cluster. "Who's the legal guardian of Cupcake here?"

All four pointed in different directions.

"Okay," I said. "So, nobody. Fabulous."

"Excuse me," Grandma Hat cut in, eyes kind and tired. "I'm her great-aunt. Foster placement, temporary until the adoption is finalized. We were supposed to meet at the daycare. I was at the bus stop when—" She nodded toward the men "—family matters erupted."

"Family matters?" Marco choked. "He left her with a drag queen named after bubble wrap."

Miss Delilah smiled honey-slow. "And somehow she was safer with me than with you at karaoke, baby."

Lenny snapped open a compact mirror, fixed a lash, and glanced at me. "If CPS shows up, I want it known that we use silk pillowcases and we read bedtime stories with voices.

Marco's voices are chaotic."

The doors hissed. CPS arrived, punctual and inevitable.

Rivera, our local caseworker, strode in wearing a navy blazer, flats that had seen some things, and a bun so tight it had weather data. She had the calm of a librarian and the eyebrows of a judge.

"Good afternoon," she said, scanning like TSA. "I'm Rivera with Child Protective Services. I'm here for—" she checked the tablet "—'Cupcake.' That better be a nickname."

"It's a state of mind," I said. "Her actual name is in your file. She's safe with me."

Rivera nodded, taking in the emotional atmosphere of the room. "Okay, friends. Who's who?"

Bad idea. Everyone spoke at once: "I'm the god-uncle—" "I'm the foster great-aunt—" "I was promised karaoke—" "I'm emotionally trafficked—"

Rivera held up a palm. Air stilled. "Let's do it this way. Names and roles, clockwise. Keep it to one sentence and no adverbs."

While she checked IDs and documents, I patched Miss

Delilah's blister with a bandage and a travel-size Neosporin I keep specifically for patients who make me laugh.

"You are an angel in sensible shoes," she told me.

"I'm a gremlin with a license," I said.

The interracial couple's whisper fight threatened to boil again when the white guy's mother FaceTimed in and started offering opinions like a bakery offers muffins. I stepped between them before 'real family' became a weapon.

"Hey," I said quietly to him, "words like 'my real family' make messes I end up mopping. Choose better ones."

He sagged. "I'm just... tired."

"She's tired too," I said, tipping my chin to his partner. "You're on the same team. Act like it. Take turns talking, with the same number of words, and no tone police. If you need a referee, I have a blood pressure cuff and a very stern eyebrow."

He gave a breath-laugh. "Deal."

Back at the main event, Rivera was methodical, kind, and had no tolerance for nonsense. She verified the great-aunt's paperwork, the in-process adoption, the daycare timeline, and the karaoke-shaped gap.

"You left a minor with a non-listed caretaker without notice," she told Marco, voice even. "That's not a criminal act by itself, but it's unwise. Your missed handoff created a safety concern and necessitated a welfare check by the police. We don't play with handoffs."

Marco's eyes filled. "I didn't mean—"

"I know," Rivera said, softer now. "Intention doesn't bandage outcomes. We're going to do this by the book. The safest place for her right now is with her approved foster guardian. You can follow up through your attorney and your case supervisor. Today is not the day for scenes. Today is the day for signatures."

Lenny raised a trembling hand. "Can we... can we say bye?

Like, a proper one? We have a routine. She likes the 'You Are Loved' song."

Rivera's face did that human thing. She nodded. "Two minutes. Quietly. Nurse?"

"Therapy room's open," I said. "And no glitter confetti in there; the robotic vacuum chokes."

In the small room with the rocking chair and the mural of woodland animals, Lenny knelt and sang, soft and shaky, a little melody that had the shape of safety. Marco's hands hovered, unsure, then folded like prayer.

The toddler—Cupcake—looked between them with solemn, old-soul eyes, then reached out and booped each of their noses like she was saving the game. She handed Lenny the empty juice box as if it were a trophy.

"Thank you," she whispered, tiny voice like a secret.

I had to cough, so I didn't cry.

Back out in the waiting room, the peanut M&Ms finally fell from the machine with a clack like a period at the end of a long sentence. Lenny stared. "The symbolism," he breathed.

Rivera finished her forms, explained the following steps, and took Cupcake's small hand. The great-aunt stood, shoulders straighter now that the world had chosen a lane for the hour.

Miss Delilah crouched to Cupcake. "You were brave. I will bring you a sparkly backpack next time, one with a zipper that doesn't argue. Okay?"

Cupcake considered this, then nodded.

As they walked toward the doors, the room hushed. I took a swig of coffee. Cold, of course.

Behind me, the interracial couple waved me over. "We did the equal-words thing," the woman said. "It helped."

He tucked a strand of hair behind her ear. "I apologized for the couch traffic."

"I accepted," she said. "But I also requested a calendar invite for all future responsibilities, like we're at work, because apparently we only take things seriously when they have a link."

"Now that," I said, "is the sexiest sentence this hospital has heard all week."

They laughed, together this time. I handed them gold star stickers I keep for adults who remember we're all human.

At the desk, Lenny and Marco hovered. Lenny spoke first. "Does it get easier? The paperwork? The waiting? The not knowing?"

"It doesn't get easier," I said. "You get stronger. And you learn to pack snacks. And you memorize the names of good caseworkers like Rivera, and good nurses like me, who will tell you the truth even when it's crunchy."

"Crunchy truth," Marco repeated, with a half-smile. "We can do crunchy. We're very into textures."

I slid the M&Ms across the counter. "Start here. And next time, text someone who can bring backup before the promise turns into a problem."

Miss Delilah winked. "If no one has told you today, you are excessively competent."

"Girl, don't make me cry at work," I said. "OSHA got rules about hydration."

She laughed, heels clicking toward the exit.

The doors hissed again. Cupcake looked back from Rivera's side; we exchanged two-finger salutes. Then she was gone.

The room exhaled. I checked the board: three earaches, one mystery rash, and a snore consult: peace, or the budget version of it.

Security smirked. "You still don't watch reality TV?" "Why would I pay to stream my own job?" I said. He grinned. "Because on TV, they cut to a commercial." "We've got coffee breaks and bandage stickers," I said.

The fluorescent lights hummed. Somewhere, a monitor beeped steadily. I took another sip and winced.

"And for the record," I muttered, "the waiting room still ain't for the weak. But it will make you kinder."

**Coach T Says:** *Life will throw you into rooms where glitter is shedding, promises are broken, and voices rise louder than reason. But underneath all the sequins and noise, there's* *always a heartbeat asking to be seen. Compassion doesn't mean cleaning up every mess—it means pausing long enough to protect the tender, to steady the small, and to remind folks that even in chaos, love still has the final word.*

*And baby, never forget: kindness sticks longer than frosting.*

# CHAPTER 6

# LOVE OUT LOUD

After a day of sequins, karaoke confessions, and CPS paperwork, I walked out of the hospital thinking I'd left the circus behind. But the truth? The real lessons weren't waiting at the nurses' station—they were staying at home. My boys, my dog, and our kitchen table had a way of reminding me that love—loud, unapologetic love—was the only thing worth clocking into after a shift like that.

When I clock out of the ED, the hospital smell follows me like a nosy neighbor. Antiseptic, burnt coffee, and powdered gloves cling to my scrubs no matter how fast I sprint to my car.

But the moment I open my front door, the air changes. It's home. Dog hair, cinnamon candles, and that faint trace of laundry I swore I'd fold yesterday.

And then—thump... skitter... sneeze!

Here comes Kody, my blind, one-legged, allergy-ridden Yorkie, wobbling toward me like a furry pirate on a mission. Tail wagging so hard I'm afraid it'll detach, sneeze spraying my shoe, voice pitched at a full-on "I own this house" bark.

Kody doesn't know he's disabled. He doesn't know people look at him with pity. He knows this is his castle, I'm his mama, and joy is his birthright.

Watching him makes me think of my boys.

I'm the proud mama of two sons who decided early that closets were for clothes, not for living. They chose to love out loud—rainbow-bright, unapologetic, and fully themselves.

When my oldest told me he was gay, it wasn't some Hollywood scene. No violins, no dramatic pause. Just:

"Hey, Ma, you know how you keep asking if I'm dating anyone?"

"Yeah..."

"Well... I am. His name's Marcus. Also, we share hoodies." That was it. A truth dropped over leftover spaghetti.

By the time my youngest told me, I was seasoned. He sat me down, eyes wide like he was confessing to a felony. "Ma, I'm gay."

I smiled. "Okay. You want chicken for dinner, or should we do tacos?"

The way his shoulders dropped told me everything. Years of bracing against rejection... gone in one sentence.

My oldest is the smooth talker—networking in the grocery line like he's running for mayor. My youngest? The quiet sniper. One look from him will cut straight through nonsense like a scalpel.

Both of them have a radar for authenticity that puts hospital monitors to shame. And they've dragged me into their world with lessons I didn't know I needed—drag brunch etiquette ("tip like you mean it"), the fine line between shade and reading (shade is casual, reading is surgical), and the sacred healing powers of Beyoncé.

I thought I was raising them. Turns out, they were raising me too—teaching me how to stand louder, love harder, and dance worse without shame.

Loving your kids is instinct. Supporting them in a world that doesn't clap for who they are? That's a skill you learn in real time.

I messed up pronouns. I once asked if "throwing shade" meant standing under a tree. (Spoiler: it doesn't.) I googled things at 2 a.m. I sat through playlists that made my ears bleed. I got corrected, rolled my eyes back, and still kept showing up.

And when family members slid in with the "but what about..." foolishness? I shut it down quicker than a Code Blue. Because the world is already loud with judgment. My voice had to be noisier—with love.

One afternoon, years ago, we stopped at a diner after shopping. My youngest was glowing with a fresh haircut—shaved sides, rainbow streaks, and proud as hell. We were waiting for burgers when I noticed a man at the booth behind us staring at us. Not curious staring. Ugly staring.

Then he muttered something. I didn't catch all of it, but I heard enough: "Boys shouldn't..." followed by a word that made my blood boil.

I could've let it go. But I turned around so fast my ponytail had an attitude.

"Sir," I said with a smile sharp enough to slice, "I don't know what kind of day you're having, but you won't be finishing it by talking about my son like that. Not in my presence. Not in his."

He stammered something about "freedom of speech."

I leaned in, elbows on his booth. "Freedom of speech is a two-way street. You're free to say it, and I'm free to make sure you understand how wrong you are. Now enjoy your coffee—quietly."

The waitress appeared like an angel, refilled his mug without a word, and gave me the tiniest nod. My boys? Grinning like I'd handed them the moon.

That moment burned into me. You can't love your kids without fearing for them. You worry if they'll come home safe. You see the stares. You feel the air tighten.

But fear didn't make me try to dim their light. Fear made me stand next to it, so it shone brighter than Kody, who lost a leg and still struts like he's the king of the balcony. Joy survives when it knows it's loved.

If you're a parent, hear me: your kids don't just need permission to be themselves. They need celebration.

Learn their world. Defend them in rooms they'll never know they were mentioned in. Love them so loudly that their fears start packing to leave.

Of course, in my house, even deep talks end with jokes. My boys roast me like it's an Olympic event. My dance moves? "Hazardous." My clapping? "Iconic... in the wrong way." And I laugh. Because this is love in my family—safe enough to tease, strong enough to stand, soft enough to hold.

The next morning, I'm back at the hospital, badge clipped, coffee steaming, ready for whatever chaos the day might throw at me. But something's different. The weight I didn't even realize I was carrying—the worry about my boys, about whether I'm doing enough, about whether love is enough—feels lighter.

Because the truth settled in sometime between Kody's welcome-home dance and my youngest's midnight text that just said "love you, mom."

Love is enough. Love out loud is everything.

And in a world that keeps trying to whisper people into hiding, sometimes the most revolutionary thing you can do is love so loudly it drowns out all the noise.

**Coach T Says:** *Your child's journey might not look like the one you pictured—but it might be more beautiful than anything you imagined. If you can love them when the world tries to dim them, they'll shine bright enough to light the way for someone else. And don't forget: your love might be the thing that saves them.*

# CHAPTER 7

# DR. HOT MESS SAVES THE DAY

The page came over the intercom at 7:58 a.m., slicing through the relative calm of the morning: "Paging Dr. Andrew Jeeter to the ED... paging Dr. Andrew Jeeter..."

Now, to anyone else, that's just a name. But to those of us who've been in the trenches long enough, Dr. Andrew Jeeter is also known as Dr. Hot Mess—the kind of provider who could save your life while simultaneously losing his car keys, his phone, and possibly his dignity.

My coffee froze halfway to my mouth. I could feel it—the storm was rolling in, and I was about to be the poor sap with the mop when the flood hit.

"Norma," said Jackson, one of our newer nurses, sliding past the desk, "you okay? You look like you just saw a ghost."

"Not a ghost," I said. "A Category Five in cargo pants."

The triage doors swung open, and in came Dr. Hot Mess like he was auditioning for the role of ER Disaster Hero. Hair doing its own thing, scrubs wrinkled enough to qualify as textured fabric, mismatched socks peeking out from under his clogs. Oh, and a pen behind one ear... and another in his hair bun.

He carried a half-empty iced coffee in one hand and a patient chart in the other. I'm convinced he writes notes while ordering lattes.

"Morning, Norma!" he called out, way too chipper. "Let's save some lives."

I muttered under my breath, "Let's try not to burn the place down in the process."

His first patient was in Room 3—a man who had clearly been at the bar all night, his breath potent enough to knock over a houseplant. He was sprawled on the gurney, clutching his stomach like he'd been shot.

"My pain's at a ten," he moaned, "and I know my rights.

Y'all owe me a steak dinner."

Dr. Hot Mess blinked. "That's... not how hospitals work." "Then bring me chicken wings," he said, dead serious.

While the doctor tried to explain that we didn't run a sports bar, I checked his vitals. Stable as a church pew. "Sir," I said,

"if you can order off a menu, you're not dying."

Room 7 wasn't much better. The patient, a wiry man in his 50s, waved me over like he had a winning lottery ticket.

"It's my appendix," he whispered. "It's moved up here." He patted his chest.

"Your appendix?"

"Yes! I Googled it. Sometimes they migrate. Mine took the elevator to my heart."

Dr. Hot Mess somehow managed to keep a straight face. "That's... not medically possible."

The man crossed his arms. "You doctors think you know everything."

We walked out, and the doctor murmured, "I think his

Google search history is trying to kill him."

We'd barely recovered when the elderly lady in Room 12 decided to get frisky. She was sweet, usually, but today? Let's say she was feeling herself.

The second Dr. Hot Mess walked in, she leaned back, adjusted her gown, and flashed the entire nursing station through the open curtain.

"Lord, put it away," I blurted, rushing over. "This is not

Mardi Gras."

She winked. "Just showing the doctor what she's working with."

Dr. Hot Mess looked like he wanted to disappear into the floor. I threw a blanket over her lap and hissed, "Save it for bingo night, Miss Ruth."

Between cases, I was charting when I heard Dr. Hot Mess mutter, "Uh-oh" from Room 5—never a good sign.

I walked in to find a teenage boy with bright purple splotches across his chest.

"I think I'm dying," he announced. "It's spreading."

Dr. Hot Mess poked the rash with a gloved finger. "That's... grape Kool-Aid."

His mother gasped. "Bobby! Did you dump your drink on yourself again?"

He looked offended. "I was bathing in it."

The doctor's face was priceless. I backed out before I laughed so hard I needed oxygen.

Half an hour later, I caught Dr. Hot Mess in a low-key argument with Dr. Sharp, one of our more... polished physicians.

"You can't just improvise treatment like this," Dr. Sharp snapped.

"It worked, didn't it?" Hot Mess shot back.

"That's not the point—medicine isn't jazz."

Hot Mess smirked. "Maybe it should be."

I slid by them with my chart, whispering to myself, "I'd buy tickets to that concert."

The next memorable case was in Room 9—a young woman holding a takeout bag in one hand and her side with the other. She'd been in a fender bender, refused the ambulance ride, but then came in when her Uber driver told her she "looked pale."

She refused to change into a gown. "I have a date after this.

I'm not taking off my outfit."

"What's the date for?" Dr. Hot Mess asked.

She looked at us like we were the crazy ones. "To meet my future husband."

I muttered, "Might want to get that CAT scan before you meet him, sis."

And then the pager went off—possible stroke in Room 14. The joking stopped instantly.

We moved fast. Dr. Hot Mess was right there, giving orders with crisp clarity, and I was already grabbing the IV kit. The air shifted; you could feel every heartbeat in the room.

"BP's dropping," I called.

"Get neuro on the line now," he said.

We worked in sync—IV placement, labs drawn, and a CT scan ordered—all in under six minutes.

It was like watching a car that's been sputtering all morning suddenly hit the freeway at ninety with no problem. This was the side of Dr. Hot Mess that reminded you why he wore the coat, even if it was wrinkled.

When the patient was wheeled to CT, I finally exhaled. We'd just bought him a real chance.

The calm barely lasted a heartbeat. We'd just rolled the stretcher through the double doors when another call erupted from triage: "Unresponsive male at the bus stop—no pulse, no ID!"

The gurney shot into the ED as if it were on fire. A middleaged man, pale and drenched in sweat, hit our trauma bay with compressions already underway.

"Norma, bag him!" Hot Mess barked, snapping into command.

I grabbed the ambu bag, adrenaline already clawing at my throat. This wasn't funny anymore. This was raw.

Hot Mess prepped to intubate, sliding the scope into place. But just as the tube passed his cords—

The man's body jerked upright. His arm shot out and clamped around Hot Mess's wrist.

The entire room froze. For a split second, it looked like a scene out of a horror movie—a lifeless patient suddenly lunging back.

The scope clattered. Hot Mess swore. One tech stumbled into the wall. I swear somebody screamed.

Then came the seizure—violent, thrashing, knocking the side rails. Instruments hit the floor like cymbals.

"Hold him!" I shouted, diving for his IV line.

Two nurses pinned his legs. A third steadied his shoulders. His eyes rolled back, his body jerking like a puppet on snapped strings.

For the first time that day, Dr. Hot Mess didn't look messy— he looked rattled and truly rattled. His hand shook as he ordered Ativan.

We pushed the med, and seconds stretched into eternities; finally, the storm eased. His muscles slackened. The monitors found a rhythm.

I realized my own knees were trembling.

Hot Mess looked at me, wide-eyed, and whispered, "That could've gone bad."

I shook my head. "It did go bad. We just wrestled it back."

The trauma bay was a wreck—scattered instruments, staff catching their breath, my glove torn open at the wrist.

And yet, life went on. Another stretcher rolled past. A monitor beeped like it had no idea we'd just stared chaos in the face.

From Room 12, Miss Ruth hollered: "If nobody brings me

Jell-O, I'm gonna code too!" I almost laughed. Almost.

Because that's the truth about this job: the world doesn't pause for your fear. It just hands you the next crisis with a smirk.

Back at the station, Hot Mess leaned on the counter. His hair was damp with sweat, his socks still mismatched, but his voice was low, steady.

"Norma... I know I drive you crazy."

I raised an eyebrow. "You? Never."

He smiled weakly. "Thanks for catching the stuff I miss."

"That's what teammates do," I said. "We make each other look less like a headline."

And for the first time, I saw it—the messy, brilliant, fallible human under all that chaos.

**Coach T Says:** *Some people are like hurricanes—you can't stop them from blowing in, but you can choose how you stand in the wind. Chaos doesn't mean failure; sometimes it means growth in disguise. Keep your feet planted, your patience steady, and remember: even the messiest people can have the most brilliant moments. And when the room tilts from comedy to terror in a heartbeat—remember this too: you're stronger than the fear that tries to rattle you.*

# CHAPTER 8

# PANDEMONIUM IN PAJAMA PANTS

The ER has a sick sense of humor. One day ends with a Code Stroke, the kind of heart-clutching scare that leaves you praying you did enough. And the very next shift? It kicks off with SpongeBob pajama pants and a Ziploc bag of hot sauce. The ER never lets you live in one emotional lane—it's a mix of grief and giggles on shuffle.

The shift was two minutes old when SpongeBob walked in. Not SpongeBob the cartoon, bless his porous little heart—but a grown man in chartreuse pajama pants printed with forty tiny SpongeBobs doing karate kicks. He strutted through the automatic doors barefoot, hospital bracelet still on from three days ago, and clutched a gallon Ziploc of hot sauce packets like it was his emotional support animal.

"Sir?" I blinked twice because my brain needed time to catch up. "Do you have an emergency?"

"I got an appointment with my destiny," he said, clutching his side. "And a kidney stone the size of a car payment."

"That's... colorful." I grabbed a triage wristband. "Let's get you checked in, cutie."

He peered over his sunglasses. "I'm keeping the pants."

"Noted," I said. "Vitals first. Shoes off, step on the scale."

He hesitated, pointing toward the waiting area. "Not in front of her."

A woman with a stroller and a lace-front wig sharp enough to slice onions scrolled her phone without even glancing at him.

"That's my ex," he whispered. "She'll post my number on Facebook."

"Sir, weighing you is for medication safety. Nobody's posting your BMI today."

"You'd be surprised," he muttered, stepping on the scale while hugging his hot sauce bag like a teddy bear.

The numbers blinked. He hissed when the blood pressure cuff tightened. "That cuff is a liar. And also, I'm keeping the pants."

I handed him a gown at the back door.

"No."

"It's hospital policy," I chirped. "We love your undersea wardrobe, but we also love access to the parts we're treating."

He tucked the gown under his arm like a free tote bag. "Doc can access my kidney without me showing my business."

"It's your flank, babe," I said. "Nobody's coming for your business. Put on the gown."

He tilted his head heavenward. "Lord, you hear this woman?"

The Lord wisely did not comment.

I parked him in Bed 16, tossed him the gown, and told him to behave. Two minutes later, I turned around and found him attempting a ninja roll into the bed, pajama waistband still clutched, gown tied around his waist like a sarong.

"I said I would wear it," he announced, triumphant.

"Sir," I sighed, hands on hips, "your arms go in the sleeves.

That's not a sarong. That's polyester with a purpose."

Meanwhile, the floor had decided to betray me. Bed 12's IV pump started screaming, Bed 10's sitter shouted, "He's trying to climb out again!" and DeShawn, the tech, skidded by with a mop.

"Spill in the hall!" he cried. "Somebody mixed apple juice and cranberry cocktail. Wide as a swimming pool!"

Q—the SpongeBob pants man—peeked out of his curtain.

"Is this the deluxe package?"

"Sir, you have no idea," I muttered.

By then, Ms. Rivera, our charge nurse, waved me over.

"Heads up. Bed 7's family is on their way. Again."

"Which family is in Bed 7 today?" I asked.

"The sweet lady with CHF," she said. "Grandson calls himself 'Darius Esquire.' He's wearing a Shein suit, so...

church voice, Norma."

"Church voice activated," I promised.

Seconds later, the door flew open. In stormed Darius, briefcase swinging like it came free with a magazine subscription.

"I am here to represent my grandmother!" he declared.

Behind him, his grandmother called out, "Baby, ask if I can have a ginger ale!"

Q snorted so loudly his hot sauce bag rattled.

Just as I was juggling Darius, Ms. Lee's sarcasm in Bed 14, and Q's sarong crisis, a monitor alarm blared. Room 3—chest pain. My stomach dropped.

I sprinted in, heart pounding, already prepping for the worst. The patient clutched his chest, face pale... until the EKG printed. Normal. Turned out he'd pulled a muscle sneezing.

Sneezing.

I exhaled, but the scare stuck to my ribs. The ER will yank your heart into your throat, then drop you back into slapstick without apology.

Back at Bed 16, Q had knotted his gown into a pretzel around his torso, still clutching the hot sauce bag like life insurance.

Before I could fix him, the fire alarm erupted. Lights flashed. Sirens wailed. Not a drill.

Every patient craned their necks to watch. Ms. Lee yelled,

"Is this because you let pajama boy roam free?"

"Probably," I admitted.

Q raised his cup of water like a toast. "Now this is deluxe."

DeShawn groaned, shoes squeaking on the juice spill. "I swear, if one more Croc slides, I'm quitting."

Sabrina, our new nurse, whispered, "What do we do?"

"Same thing we always do," I said. "Keep patients calm, keep ourselves calmer, and pray nobody bolts for the parking lot."

As if on cue, Mr. Romano was halfway down the hall before Kayla tackled him like an NFL linebacker.

By the time the alarms finally stopped, the hall smelled like fruit punch and fear. Q was tucked back in bed with his gown half on, and my Fitbit thought I'd run a 5K.

"You know," Q said, smirking, "if you'd just let me keep the sarong, I'd behave."

I laughed. "Sir, you've been here forty minutes and caused more drama than most people manage in a week."

He grinned. "I aim to please."

**Coach T Says:** *Some days in the ER feel like a slapstick comedy you never auditioned for. Pajama pants roll in, alarms sing in four-part harmony, and somebody always spills something you end up mopping in Crocs.*

*But here's the truth: You can't control every mess. What you can control is how you show up in it.*

*So, laugh when you can. Breathe when you must. And baby, remember this—sometimes the only thing holding it all together is the same thing keeping that gown on: one good knot.*

# CHAPTER 9

# SUNDAY DINNER AND SIDE-EYE

Sundays were supposed to be my day off. A day to rest, recharge, maybe even put my feet up. Instead, they had somehow evolved into a weekly production where my kitchen turned into a food truck without wheels, and my dining room became a low-stakes casino for 50¢ a card.

It always started the same: me swearing under my breath that I wasn't doing this again—while preheating the oven, seasoning chicken, and wiping down counters I'd just cleaned the night before. I moved like a short-order cook in an apron that had survived more grease splatters than any one piece of fabric should.

By 9 a.m., the first pot was already simmering—collard greens slow-cooking with smoked turkey legs. The smell was a warm, savory hug, the kind that could drag neighbors in from two blocks over. By 9:30, the macaroni and cheese was in the oven, and the cornbread batter was ready to pour. A ham glazed in pineapple rings was waiting for its oven time, and I had a mental countdown running for the fried chicken rotation, as if I were directing air traffic.

I'd tried "scaling down" once. That was the year I served spaghetti and garlic bread, thinking I'd save myself the hassle. Instead, I got three phone calls asking if I was sick, two knocks on my door with store-bought pies "just in case," and one very disappointed look from an older neighbor who told me, "Baby, that ain't Sunday dinner."

I didn't invite all these people. Not exactly. It started years ago with "Come over for Sunday dinner" to a few close friends and cousins. Now it was "Norma's house is open on Sundays," which apparently meant anyone with a distant connection and a sturdy appetite could wander in.

At 10:15, my phone buzzed with the first warning. We're bringing company, the text read. No name. No context. Just the universal Sunday Dinner code to prepare yourself.

The first interruption came before the chicken even hit the skillet. My neighbor Earl, who "happened to be in the area," dropped by to "return" a Tupperware from two weeks ago—conveniently timed so he could sniff the air and ask what I was cooking. I handed him a deviled egg and sent him on his way before he could angle for a full plate.

By noon, my front door had swung open at least six times. No one knocked. No one rang. A breeze of perfume, hair grease, and outside air wafted in with each arrival. First through the door was a neighbor named Clarice, wearing heels in my house as if she were walking a runway between the living room and kitchen.

"I brought sweet tea," she announced, holding up a gallon jug that was sweating harder than a politician in July. "And

I might have invited a friend from my choir."

I raised an eyebrow. "The soprano or the bass?"

She grinned. "Yes."

Ten minutes later, the choir friend (bass) arrived with a buddy named Rico, who had a smile that made me wonder if he was trying to sell me something. Behind them came two local teens carrying folding chairs and the giant plastic bin I knew held our bingo supplies.

"Where do you want the chairs?" one of the teens asked.

"Anywhere that's not blocking my path to the stove," I said, dodging around them with a tray of cornbread.

By 2 p.m., the table was groaning under the weight of food, and the dining room was buzzing. The ham glistened, the fried chicken was stacked like golden bricks of currency, and the macaroni cheese had that perfect crust you could hear crack when the spoon went in.

Sunday dinner was an event. A production. A Broadway show with gravy. People lined up buffet-style, plates clattering, side-eye exchanged over the last chicken wing. Everyone knew the rule: eat first, play later.

Bingo didn't start until after dessert, but the trash talk started at the first bite.

"I'm telling you right now," Clarice said, sliding into her seat with a plate that could've fed three, "I'm taking the pot today. Y'all better have my quarters ready."

"You couldn't win if you had the answers taped to your forehead," fired back Miss Geraldine, an older woman from down the block with an afro puff so perfect it could be in a museum.

By the time dessert hit the table—banana pudding, peach cobbler, pound cake—the competitive energy had reached a low simmer. Rico strolled over to the bingo bin like he was walking into Vegas.

Cards were 50¢ each. I kept a mason jar for the quarters, and when it hit the table, it was like a bell at the start of a boxing match.

Rico, the new guy, bought five cards right off the bat. Clarice narrowed her eyes. "Oh, you think you're a big spender, huh?"

"I came to win," Rico said with a grin.

The first game was smooth—B-12, G-46, O-71—until I called "N-33" and Miss Geraldine yelled "Bingo!" so loud my dog jumped. She collected the $6 pot with a smirk, and I swear she winked at Rico like it was personal.

By the third game, things got heated. The choir friend accused Clarice of double-marking. Clarice accused him of "breathing too loudly on her board." Meanwhile, Rico quietly racked up two wins, and by the time we got to blackout, he'd cleared $9.50 in quarters.

"Y'all let the new guy rob us blind," Clarice huffed, crossing her arms.

"That's called skill," Rico said.

In the middle of the fifth game, someone knocked over a glass of sweet tea, soaking three cards and prompting an argument over whether they could be replaced for free. I settled it by handing over fresh cards with a warning that

"sticky numbers are not my problem."

I was in the kitchen loading plates into the sink when I heard someone behind me. It was one of the teens who'd brought the chairs. She hesitated, twisting a quarter in her fingers.

"I, uh... just wanted to say thanks," she mumbled.

"For what, baby?" I asked, turning from the sink.

"For this. For Sundays. My mom works a lot, and... we don't really do stuff like this at home. I know it's just bingo, but it's fun." She shrugged. "Feels like family."

I smiled, suddenly glad for every pot I'd scrubbed and

every ham I'd glazed. "Well, you are family now. You hear me? Bring your mama next time."

She nodded, and for a second, the noise of the bingo crowd faded into the background.

By the time the last game wrapped up, the table looked like a war zone, the cornbread was reduced to crumbs, and my kitchen resembled a scene that raccoons had ransacked. I collected the leftover cards and the jar of quarters (minus

$19.50 in winnings), and then collapsed into a chair.

Clarice flopped down across from me. "Same time next week?"

I groaned. "Y'all gonna be the death of me."

"Yeah," she said, smirking. "But at least you'll be well-fed." And she wasn't wrong.

**Coach T Says:** *Home isn't just where you hang your hat—it's where the gravy stains live, where the side-eye is fluent, and where someone's always ready to take your last chicken wing and your bingo money.*

*You don't need a perfect house or a perfect meal to create a tradition worth keeping. Sometimes all it takes is a kitchen*

*full of noise, a table full of mismatched chairs, and a community that shows up—whether you invite them or not.*

*Laugh at the chaos, love the people, and remember... those 50¢ bingo pots buy more joy than you think.*

# CHAPTER 10

# THE SHIFT THAT WOULDN'T END

If Sunday fed my soul with gravy and bingo cards, Monday tried to starve it with beeps and bed alarms. The plan was innocent. Naïve, even. I would float onto the unit for a quick eight, keep my head down, dodge any "special projects," and leave on time with my dignity, my edges, and my ankles intact.

The universe laughed.

"Norma," the unit secretary said, handing me the census with the solemnity of a will reading, "we're at capacity plus guests."

"Guests?" I asked.

"People who arrived with other people and never left," she said. "They have snacks."

The hallway already sounded like a percussion section—call bells pinging, pumps chiming, monitors clearing their throats dramatically. A resident hurried past, reading a chart as if it were bad news in tiny font. Housekeeping parked a yellow "Wet Floor" sign exactly where everyone would ignore it.

"Short eight," I muttered to myself, tying my hair up tighter. "We believe in the fiction. We live the lie."

My assignment lit up the screen: four patients and two admits "arriving shortly," which is hospital speak for "surprise."

Room 214 was first. The door was cracked; a Styrofoam cup sat on the ledge, as if it were supervising. Inside, a woman in her forties—eyes red, posture squared—clutched a Tupperware of soup like a relic. Her husband lay in bed, propped up, more gray than yesterday.

"Hi, I'm Norma," I said softly.

She glanced at my badge, then at me, as if confirming I was real. "I made his favorite. Chicken and rice. I brought a spoon."

The patient stirred, gave me a tired half-smile. "She cooks like she's feeding an army."

"Lucky army," I said. "Let me check with dietary and the doc; we'll see what's safe."

She nodded, but her eyes were already asking the question beneath the spoon. I looked at the drip, the oxygen, and the chart glowing from the wall computer. I knew what the med notes said. I also knew that none of the notes spoke her language yet.

"Give me five minutes," I said. "Then we talk about eating... and everything else."

Across the hall, 212's call light pinged with the impatient kind of ding that says I know you heard me. I stepped in to find an older man with a stubborn jaw and the alertness of someone who had slept with one eye open, even before the advent of monitors.

"Sir?" I asked.

He folded his arms. "An angel visited me last night."

"Okay," I said, neutral. "And what did the angel say?"

He pointed at the IV pump. "Said I shouldn't take that."

"Well," I said, glancing at the antibiotic with a name that ends in "-cin," as if it meant business, "did the angel have a pharmacy license?"

He cracked a smile.

Down the hall, a new nurse brushed past with the thousandyard stare of someone who'd just met her first "I have to go now" and lost. She ducked into the supply closet, and the door clicked shut with a please don't follow me finality.

I followed her anyway.

She had her back against the shelves, mascara smudged like it had survived a tiny hurricane. "I missed a med time. I charted in the wrong place. I asked a patient if they wanted grape or orange juice, and it was an NPO order. I'm a disaster."

"You're a nurse," I said, which is both an answer and a diagnosis. "Rule one: you're allowed one private cry per shift, but not in the bathroom because somebody will knock.

Supply closet tears don't count toward your limit."

She laughed through the clog in her throat.

"You're going to get feedback," I said. "We all do. You'll say, 'Thank you,' and then you'll come back tomorrow and do five things right you didn't know how to do today. That's the job."

Virgil poked his head in, mask slipped for a second while he swallowed coffee. "Are we doing closet coaching?" "We do coaching wherever it fits," I said.

"Need me to stall anybody?"

"Yes," I said. "Everyone."

By noon, my "short eight" had become an "unexpected twelve." The attending wrote orders in prose length; the printer jammed in three languages; transport was "on the way" across two time zones.

I got 212 to agree to the antibiotic after explaining what bacteria do when they think you're bluffing. I told 214's wife the truth that no one wanted to say out loud, and then sat with her while she finally came to terms with it. We spooned a tiny bit of broth to her husband's lips. He closed his eyes like it was church.

By evening, the unit glowed the color of microwaved dinners and fluorescent resolve. The new nurse came bouncing out of Room 210 like she'd just won a marathon. "Two wins," she said. "Vitals recheck and a perfect IV flush."

"As you should," I said. "Take your victory lap in the med room."

My feet ached, a particular ache that no pedometer respects. The elevator dinged like mercy.

Virgil caught me at the exit. "Eat with people. You look like you're about to dine on a vending machine dinner that will not nourish your soul."

"I have granola in my bag," I said.

"That," he said, "is exactly what I mean. Come on. Two blocks over. Good lasagna. People who don't beep."

The transition from hospital to dinner felt like stepping through a portal. One moment, I was surrounded by monitors and antiseptics; the next, I was walking through a neighborhood where porch lights glowed a warm yellow, and the air smelled like someone's grandmother was cooking.

The apartment belonged to a friend of Virgil's: a low ceiling fan, soft lights, and a plant that had survived three owners by sheer will. The table—scarred wood, family-sized—was already crowded with mismatched plates and a lasagna the size of a carry-on.

"Norma," said the host, apron dusted with marinara constellations, "we've heard legends. Sit. We feed legends."

"Careful," I said. "I'm only heroic every other Tuesday."

The first bite felt like someone had whispered 'shhh' to my nervous system. The second bite reminded me I hadn't sat all day except to hover at bedsides, which isn't sitting so much as standing politely with knees.

And then it happened. You put a nurse at a table, and the stories start looking for you.

A teenager with a high ponytail and a college brochure under her elbow cleared her throat. "Is it normal to choose a major and immediately hate yourself?"

A cousin with perfect nails stared into her water. "Is it normal to feel like you failed because your marriage didn't?"

At the end of the table, a woman with a headscarf whispered, "Is it normal to be mad at everyone who texts 'let me know what you need' because you don't know what you need?"

Every head turned toward me as if I'd brought a syllabus.

Virgil sipped his wine and gave me the go-ahead look.

"I'm off-duty," I said, which made precisely no difference.

So I set my fork down and made a circle out of a rectangle.

"Ground rules. No interrupting. No fixing. Questions start with 'What' or 'How,' not 'Why.' If you cry, someone hands you a napkin, not a solution. Deal?"

They nodded. The radio found a softer station.

The teen admitted she wasn't afraid of failing classes so much as disappointing a counselor who called her "our star." The cousin said she felt like she'd broken a contract, and we discussed how sometimes keeping your promises to yourself means breaking the ones that are hurting you. The woman with the headscarf said her phone dinged like a slot machine after chemo, and she wanted to throw it in the freezer.

Nobody fixed anything. But the air shifted—lighter, kinder. Someone passed bread without asking. Someone refilled my water without me noticing. We laughed, too. Virgil told the story of a bed alarm that refused to be reasonable. I mentioned a patient who once paid me in candy bars for untangling his cords—"reparations for tubing wranglers."

At some point, a small pad of paper appeared next to my plate. Without meaning to, I wrote three words: emotional first aid. Then I drew a crooked box around them like they might run away if I looked away.

When I finally stood to go, the host hugged me with one arm so she wouldn't soil my scrubs. "You come back. Every time you do, people leave breathing easier."

On the sidewalk, the night was the good kind of quiet—the hush that follows a day that did not defeat you.

Virgil walked beside me. "You turned dinner into group therapy," he teased.

"I didn't," I said. "The table did."

We reached the corner where our paths split. He saluted.

"See you tomorrow, Coach."

Back home, my kitchen was a still life of my life: soaking pots, leftover containers, a bingo card shoved under a cookbook. I set my bag down and pulled the note from my pocket.

Emotional first aid.

Under it, I wrote: TECU? Then, small in the corner, like a secret: The Emotional Check-Up.

I stuck it on the fridge with a tomato magnet. It looked silly and serious at the same time. So do most new things.

I turned off the light, and the kitchen exhaled. The day was over. The work wasn't. It never is.

I didn't know it yet, but that crooked little note would outlive the shift. It would become a map.

**Coach T says:** *Some shifts won't end when the clock says they should. They'll follow you home, sit at your table, and stare you down until you admit what they already know: your gift isn't just starting IVs—it's starting conversations that let people breathe again.*

If that's you, try this:

- Make a circle out of a rectangle. Any table can be a place to heal if you set ground rules.
- Don't fix—hand napkins. Presence matters more than solutions.
- Write down the whisper. If an idea keeps tapping your shoulder, give it a name, even if it's messy.

TECU doesn't start in a boardroom. It begins in the quiet after the beeps, where you decide your voice matters—on and off the unit.

The next morning brought the kind of chaos that makes you question your life choices before your first sip of coffee. The day picked a fight with me before I even got out of the driveway.

I was already running late—hair halfway pinned, coffee in a travel mug that tasted like hope—when I saw it. My car leaned at a pitiful angle, as if it had just given up on life. Flat. Not one tire. Not two. All four, slashed clean like somebody auditioned for Fast & Furious: Petty Edition.

"Lord," I muttered, setting my mug on the hood, "give me strength not to flip out before 7 a.m."

That's when I noticed the note flapping under my wiper.

Written in Sharpie, letters big and angry: "IF I CAN'T HAVE

YOU, SHE DAMN SURE CAN'T."

I froze. "Uh... excuse me?"

I scanned the lot like I expected the masked avenger to pop out from behind the dumpsters. Instead, I spotted my neighbor Troy, stumbling out in basketball shorts, squinting at his own car like it had personally betrayed him.

"Norma," he called, scratching his head, "what happened to your ride?"

I pointed at the note. "Apparently, I'm in a love triangle I didn't sign up for."

Before he could respond, blue and red lights pulled into the lot. A patrol car parked crooked, and out stepped Officer Sanchez, sipping gas-station coffee and looking like this was not her first round of neighborhood nonsense.

She crouched by my shredded tires, then held up the note with two gloved fingers. "This yours?"

"Do I look like the kind of woman who writes angry ransom notes to myself?" I said, hands on hips.

Sanchez smirked. "Fair." She clicked her pen. "Any enemies, exes, or jealous spouses we should know about?"

"Ma'am," I said flatly, "I don't even have time to fold my laundry. I promise you nobody's fighting over me."

That's when the building manager waddled over, clutching a tablet. "Caught it on the security feed," he announced, already sweating. "Drunk woman in a ski mask. She staggered up, cursed at the car window, then stabbed the tires like she was in a slasher film. After she stomped off, she tripped over her own purse."

I blinked. "And let me guess—wrong car?"

Troy groaned, burying his face in his hands. "Yeah. Mine.

One of my... uh... situations."

"Situations?" I repeated, arms crossed.

Officer Sanchez raised a brow. "You mean one of your mistresses."

Troy winced. "Don't use the M-word."

I pointed at my ruined tires. "Sir, she used the K-word—knife."

The officer chuckled, jotting notes. "Well, at least it's a case of mistaken identity. I'll file it as criminal mischief, but good luck explaining this to your insurance."

I sighed, staring at my poor car like it had been drafted into someone else's soap opera. "So I'm late for work, stranded, and apparently starring in Real Housewives of DC Apartments. Fabulous."

Troy shuffled closer, sheepish. "Look, Norma, I'm sorry. I'll pay for the tires. She wasn't supposed to come by."

"Clearly she came by and brought props," I snapped. "Handle your drama, Troy. My scrubs don't come with a side of tire slashing."

Just then, another patrol car rolled up, lights still spinning. A rookie officer stepped out, notebook ready. "Dispatch said we got a domestic?"

I threw my hands up. "More like a Domino's—because everything keeps falling and I'm the pizza that got dropped."

The rookie blinked. Officer Sanchez snorted into her

coffee.

Troy groaned louder.

By the time the report was filed, my shift had already started.

I called an Uber, clutching my travel mug like a lifeline. As we pulled away, and I watched my poor car slumped in the lot, tires sagging like it was too tired to keep secrets.

The driver glanced at me in the rearview. "Rough morning?" I laughed the kind of laugh that's mostly air. "You don't even know. And I still gotta go save lives looking like I lost a fight with a soap opera villain."

The hospital doors came into view. I squared my shoulders, pasted on my "don't try me" smile, and thought, 'If this is the pre-show, Lord, help me with the main event."

**Coach T Says:** *Sometimes life slashes your tires before you even get started. But how you handle the chaos—with grace, boundaries, and a refusal to let someone else's drama define your day—that's where your real strength shows. Keep your shoulders squared and your smile ready. The world needs what you bring to it, flat tires and all.*

# CHAPTER 11

# FLAT TIRES, FULL SHIFT

I knew the day was going to be messy the moment my phone lit up with 27 unread messages before 8 a.m. Family Group Chat—Momma Bell's Family Dinner THIS SUNDAY—Mandatory Attendance.

Mandatory, my ass. I love my family, but they throw

"mandatory" around like they're the CDC and I'm Patient Zero.

The messages kept pinging:

- "Norma, bring your sweet potato pie."
- "Norma, wear something nice—no scrubs this time."
- "Norma, don't be late like last Easter."

I sipped my coffee... and nearly gagged—lukewarm hazelnut sludge. Somebody hadn't cleaned the machine since the Bush administration. Perfect start.

By the time I walked into the ER, the waiting room was already a zoo: toddlers screaming in harmony, a man in camo asleep across three chairs, and a volunteer trying to explain to an older woman, why her cat couldn't be seen in the trauma bay.

I paused at the double doors and checked my armor: badge, pens, trauma shears, ChapStick, and patience, which I would definitely see tested. The ER smell hit as the doors whooshed open—antiseptic, burnt coffee, and floor cleaner that had clearly lost the fight.

And then came the music: call bells pinging, pumps chiming, monitors sighing like they were over it. A resident sprinted past, eyes glued to a chart. Housekeeping parked a "Wet Floor" sign directly in the busiest hallway.

"Short eight," I muttered, tying my hair tighter. "We believe in the fiction. We live the lie."

"Norma!" my charge nurse barked before I could even find my locker. "Chest pain in Bay 3, slip-and-fall in 4, and a guy in 6 holding... something wet."

I rounded the corner and met Wet Guy.

He beamed at me, holding a mason jar filled with cloudy brown liquid. "This is my mama's soup," he declared. "She's been sick since she ate it. I figured you folks could, you know, test it."

blinked. "Sir, this is an ER, not CSI: Chicken Noodle."

Before he could argue, another voice slid in smooth as silk. "Norma Jean Woods?"

I turned—petite frame, perfect brows, hair in a no-nonsense bun, confidence rolling off her like perfume. "Nurse Mai," she said, shaking my hand. "Heard about you."

"All lies, I hope."

She smirked. "Depends who you ask."

Within minutes, we were tag-teaming like we'd trained together. She was crisp, fast, efficient—the kind of nurse who could juggle three IVs and still walk away with her edges intact. Chest pain guy calmed under her steady rhythm, slip-and-fall lady tried flirting with her, and Wet Guy hovered in the hallway like we were denying his jar a baptism.

"Chain of custody," I told him, slipping the jar into the

biohazard bin. "You give it to me, I give it to the bin, the bin gives it to the underworld."

Sixty percent of nursing is timing.

As we worked, my phone buzzed again.

Mai raised a brow. "Your boyfriend blowing you up?"

snorted. "Worse. My family. They think I can drop everything for Sunday dinner."

"They guilt-trip you?"

"Girl, I'm lucky if I pee during a shift. The only Sunday plan

I've got is sweatpants and ignoring everybody."

She chuckled. "Vietnamese moms do emotional terrorism. Mine texts me pictures of empty chairs when I miss Sunday lunch."

I nodded, impressed. "Respect."

She smirked. "Just wait till you meet my brother."

Around noon, she popped her head into the supply. "My brother's dropping off my lunch. You want anything?"

"I've got vending machine almonds."

Her face said my snack had offended her ancestors.

Five minutes later, I heard it. A voice at the nurses' station.

Smooth. Confident. "I've got lunch for Mai."

I looked up. And Lord help me.

Tall. Shoulders like a linebacker. Smile like a secret. Eyes the color of melted espresso.

"You must be Norma," he said.

blinked. "Depends who's asking."

"Norma," Mai cut in, smirking, "this is my brother, Khai."

He leaned just close enough for me to catch the scent of clean soap and cedar. "Nice wig," he said with a grin.

I froze. "Excuse me?"

"I notice details," he shrugged. "Looks good."

Somebody down the hall whispered, "Get it, Norma." I wanted to melt into the floor.

Khai slid a container across to Mai. "Pork belly, pickled vegetables, extra rice. And chopsticks... in case your vending almonds are tired of being disrespected."

I opened my mouth to say something slick. Instead: "I... like rice."

Lord, take my badge.

His grin deepened. "Good. Maybe I'll bring enough for two next time."

And then he walked away, his posture perfect, leaving me holding a smile I hadn't authorized.

Before my brain could process Khai's smile, the intercom blared: "Code Blue—Room 7."

Shift over. Game face on.

We hit the room fast: CPR, meds, chaos. Soup Guy even wandered in, like a side quest I hadn't ordered.

"Sir," I snapped, "unless your soup can do compressions, get out!"

Mai and I worked in sync—compressions, meds, defib. My

arms burned, my lungs begged, and still we pushed. Finally, a pulse. Borrowed, but real.

The relief was sharp. The kind that makes your hands tremble when you try to hold a water cup.

I stepped into the hallway. Soup Guy clutched his jar. "So... no testing?"

"Sir," I said flatly, "if you love your mama, throw that soup out and order her a sandwich."

For once, he nodded.

By the end of the shift, I was wrung out—scrubs sticking, patience paper-thin, feet screaming. The gossip mill had already nicknamed me and Khai "Khnorma." Someone taped it to my water bottle. I pretended to be annoyed.

But when I drove home, quiet at last, the truth hit me like a brick:

I'd saved a life, juggled chaos, laughed with Mai, and been looked at by a man like I was more than my badge. And yet...

I was still bone-deep empty.

I gripped the wheel harder. I can't keep this pace forever.

Even the thought of family dinner felt like another shift I didn't clock into. Not because I didn't love them—but because love doesn't refill you if you're already running on fumes.

That night, I sat at my kitchen table, still in half-damp scrubs, staring at a blank index card. My pen tapped until the words spilled: TECU—the Emotional Check-Up.

I looked at it, heart thudding. I realized that I'd been conducting emotional check-ups throughout my career. For patients. For families. For new nurses crying in closets. But never for myself.

The card pulsed at me from the fridge like it knew.

**Coach T Says:** *Even in the middle of the mess—codes, chaos, and soup jars—you're still a whole person. Don't* *forget her. She's worth saving, too.*

# CHAPTER 12

# THE HOSPITAL AT FULL TILT

The sign-up sheet appeared like contraband on the break room fridge at 6:12 a.m.

POTLUCK WEDNESDAY -- BRING A DISH, BRING A FORK, BRING NO DRAMA.

Someone had added in different handwriting: (Lies. Bring drama.)

By 9:30, the table was a United Nations of carbs. Aluminum pans steamed, crockpots blinked one suspicious red eye, and the room smelled like cumin met brown sugar and made a truce. Labels were generous at best: Jollof-ish, Lumpia (yes, fried), Mac & Cheese (respect the crust), Ghost-Pepper Goat (NOT KIDDIE SAFE), Banana Pudding (fight me).

"Who brought the ghost-pepper goat?" I asked, fanning my face with a glove box.

"My auntie," an RT confessed. "She said if you cry, you're welcome."

"Solid metric," I said. "I'll alert Chaplaincy."

Our charge nurse planted hands on hips. "Norma, you're the hot-food guard. No stampedes."

"I run triage, not a buffet."

"Same skill set," she said. "Prioritize, prevent chaos, keep the peace."

She wasn't wrong.

At 11:40, we opened the floodgates. "Line starts on the left," I announced, wielding tongs like a marshal. "One protein, one starch, one wild card. Clean your own mess. Amen."

Mai breezed in with bánh mì like a benevolent queen. "Spicy mayo separate. I love you, but not enough to chart your heartburn."

The first warning sign came at 12:07—a rad tech sprinted

past, gasping, "Ghost-pepper goat! Whooooo!" Second sign at 12:11—same tech, red and sweating. "Ghost-pepper goat... help."

I handed him milk like absolution. He chugged repentance.

Then came the visitor. Gym-fit, don't-test-me posture. He piled goat high, added jollof, two lumpia, and "one of everything for fairness." First bite, he grinned. "I don't feel anything—"

Hiccup. Sweat broke like rain—eyes watering.

"You good?" I asked, angling him into a chair.

"Hot," he croaked. "Like... Satan's bathtub."

Mai slid milk across like a card shark. "Small sips. Don't prove a point. Prove you want to live."

That's when a shadow filled the doorway. Expensive tie. Shoes that screamed orthopedic money. Medical Director, energy radiating five feet in every direction.

Virgil's father. My stomach dropped.

"I heard there is an... unsanctioned meal event," he said.

The room froze mid-chew.

"Doctor," I said with my best church-usher smile, "this is a cultural appreciation morale initiative. No open flames, allergens labeled, sanitizer flowing, food far from patient care."

He surveyed the spread like a general reviewing troops. A single nostril flicker betrayed him. His eyes did a quick lap—jollof, goat, bánh mì, mac, banana pudding.

"Potlucks require managerial notification," he said carefully.

"Of course," I said. "Next time we'll CC seventeen people."

"Given that today is Wing Day in the cafeteria, an exception may be made."

From the coffee machine, someone whispered, "He hates

Wing Day."

I plated a diplomat's sampler. He took one careful bite of goat. Blink. Tilt. A single dignified tear. "Acceptable. In moderation."

I boxed banana pudding "for policy review." He cleared his throat to cover his joy. "Email your... coordinator notes." "Subject line: Morale Works Better Than Wings," I said.

"We'll workshop the title."

He left pretending he wasn't delighted. We exhaled as a group.

The calm lasted exactly seven minutes.

"CODE BLUE—BAY TWO."

Plates down. Mask up. We moved.

Bay Two: middle-aged man, mid-sentence collapse. CPR started. Meds flying. The code cart drawers slid like slot machines. Mai grabbed the crash cart while I started compressions.

"Pulse!" someone called after what felt like forever—borrowed, faint, but real.

Before we could catch our breath: "TRAUMA ALERT—

ETA THREE MINUTES."

The trauma bay exploded into controlled chaos. Motor vehicle accident rolled in—lacerated scalp, tender chest, left forearm bent wrong. We cut clothes, started IVs, and got Xrays moving. The patient kept asking about his dog while trying not to howl when his arm reminded him of physics.

"Your phone?" I said. "We'll call anyone you need."

That's when the overhead chimed again: "ETA TWO—

GUNSHOT WOUND WALK-IN."

Walk-in. Because why not?

He staggered through doors with a friend and a story that changed twice: Through-and-through thigh, bleeding contained by bravado and a belt that shouldn't be used for tourniquets. We moved him to Bay Six, traded the belt for real pressure, called surgery, called the part of ourselves that refuses to be jaded.

Between cases, I split myself the way good nurses do. Trauma bay—vitals, pain meds, consent explained like a human, not a form. Gunshot stabilized; the kid tried to smile; I wiped away a tear he didn't ask me to see.

The wave finally broke around 5:40 p.m. The board showed fewer red flags. The potluck table sat empty, smelling faintly of curry, bleach, and something sweet.

I washed my hands like I could erase adrenaline and walked one last loop. Trauma patient sleeping through pain-controlled rest, arm splinted neatly. Gunshot kid stared at the ceiling, jaw unclenched. I stood there long enough to be a person, not a badge. "You're safe for the moment."

He blinked hard and nodded.

Back at the desk, under the keyboard, a bright sticky note waited: TECU—just letters, but louder than a page.

Mai leaned beside me. "You looked somewhere else for a second."

"I was," I said. "A table. Any table. No wristbands. Still... healing."

She tapped the sticky. "You've been doing it in hallways for years."

As I clocked out, I passed the dark break room and shut off the light. Outside, my scrubs still carried the scent of jollof and bleach, borrowed time and something like hope.

I listened for phantom beeps and heard, just under them, the whisper I'd been ignoring: Why am I only allowed to heal inside these walls?

**Coach T Says:** *Community is a vital sign. Feed it and it feeds you back. When chaos hits, remember: shared tables create shared strength. Label the heat, stagger the line, sit with the waiting. That's how cultures change—one potluck, one steady pair of hands, one whispered plan for healing beyond the beeps.*

# CHAPTER 13

# CONVERSATIONS THAT CUT DEEPER

The day had already flexed its crazy muscles before sunrise. Triage was a circus, the monitors were screaming like a choir, and I was one coffee away from baptizing myself in hazelnut creamer.

But it was Room 18 that stopped me in my tracks.

Inside sat a wiry man in his late fifties, his hospital gown tied half-heartedly, like it was daring someone to fix it. His eyes carried that mix of "I've seen too much" and "I'm not telling you half of it." His chart screamed CHF exacerbation; his soul whispered something else entirely.

"Morning," I said, pulling up a chair instead of standing with the clipboard armor. "How's your breathing?" He gave a half-smile. "Better than my marriage." Well, damn.

I leaned back, smirking. "We don't carry meds for that one."

He chuckled, then his face cracked into something raw. "You ever stay in something long past its expiration date?"

My gut tightened. Divorce. Split holidays. Custody calendars. My own reflection nodded back at me. "Yeah," I said softly. "Sometimes you stay because leaving feels scarier than bleeding."

The room went quiet. The heart monitor ticked like a metronome.

"I thought if I stayed, I was strong," he admitted. "Turns out,

I was just scared."

I felt that one in my chest. Not the patient chart kind of chest pain, but the soul ache—the one that nudged me closer to the path I hadn't fully stepped on yet. Coaching. Guiding and helping people untangle the emotional mess that no IV could fix.

"You're not weak for walking away," I told him, voice steady. "You're human. Sometimes healing means disappointing the version of you that thought you could endure it all."

He blinked, slowly. Then whispered, "That's the first thing that's made sense in months."

I sat with him. No alarms. No interruptions. Just two people, sharing the kind of medicine you don't chart.

The rest of the shift bled into its usual mess—Virgil cracking jokes at the desk, Ms. Betty stealing graham crackers from the supply cart, Dr. Hot Mess tripping on his stethoscope again. But I carried Room 18 with me like a secret.

The next morning brought the kind of shift that makes you question your life choices before your first sip of coffee. I was assigned to the cardiac unit, which meant pacemakers, bypass recoveries, and the kind of chest pain that keeps everyone awake at night.

Room 302 was Mr. Davidson, post-op day two from a triple bypass. His wife sat in the corner chair like a sentinel, knitting needles clicking in rhythm with his heart monitor.

"How's he doing?" she asked without looking up from her

stitches.

"Steady," I said, checking his surgical site. "Healing takes time."

She nodded, but I caught the tremor in her hands. " Fortythree years," she said quietly. "We've been married fortythree years. I don't know how to do this alone."

Mr. Davidson stirred, eyes fluttering open. "You won't have to," he whispered, voice hoarse from the breathing tube. "I'm not going anywhere, Ruth."

She finally looked up, tears spilling over her reading glasses. "You promised me that before, Harold. Right before the heart attack in the grocery store."

The air in the room shifted. This wasn't just about medical recovery—this was about trust rebuilt one heartbeat at a time.

"Mrs. Davidson," I said, pulling up the second chair, "what's the scariest part for you?"

She set down her knitting, hands shaking. "The not knowing. When he clutches his chest, is it gas or is it goodbye? When he's quiet too long, is he resting or...?" She couldn't finish.

Mr. Davidson reached for her hand, the one with the wedding ring worn thin. "Ruth, look at me."

She did, reluctantly.

"I'm going to learn to take my pills. I'm going to walk every morning. I'm going to stop eating bacon like it's a food group." He squeezed her fingers. "But I need you to stop watching me like I'm already dead."

The monitors beeped their steady rhythm while they stared at each other across a chasm of fear and forty-three years of love.

"What would help you both feel safer?" I asked.

They looked at me like I'd asked them to solve calculus.

"I mean it," I continued. "Not what the discharge planner says. What would actually help you sleep at night?"

Mr. Davidson spoke first. "I want to know what warning signs are real and which ones are just... life."

"I want to stop being terrified every time he goes to the bathroom," Mrs. Davidson added.

We spent the next twenty minutes discussing the differences between everyday recovery aches and red-flag symptoms. I taught her how to take his pulse—strong and steady—and showed her breathing exercises that didn't require a trip to the ER.

When I left their room, they were sitting closer, her knitting abandoned, his color better than it had been all morning.

Room 308 held a different kind of heartbreak. Maria Santos, twenty-eight years old, had postpartum cardiomyopathy. Her heart was failing three weeks after giving birth to her first child.

Her mother sat beside the bed, holding a sleeping baby, while Maria stared at the ceiling.

"She won't hold him," her mother whispered to me. "She says she's afraid she'll hurt him."

I approached Maria's bedside carefully. "How are you feeling today?"

"Like my body betrayed me," she said without looking away from the ceiling tiles. "I carried him for nine months. I did everything right. And now my heart is broken—literally broken—and I can't even trust myself to hold my own son."

The baby stirred in grandmother's arms, making those soft newborn sounds that usually melt hearts. Maria's eyes filled, but she didn't reach for him.

"What if I collapse while holding him? What if my heart stops and he falls?" Her voice cracked. "What if I'm not meant to be his mother?"

I sat on the edge of her bed, careful not to disturb the monitor wires. "Maria, your heart is healing. Your body is healing.

But your mind is still in emergency mode."

She finally looked at me. "How do you know?"

"Because I've seen fear dress up as protection. And right now, you're trying to protect your baby from you—but what he needs is to feel your heartbeat, even if it's not perfect." Her mother leaned forward. "Mija, you are his mother. Sick or well, scared or brave—you're his mother."

"What's one small thing you could do to connect with him without feeling unsafe?" I asked.

Maria thought for a long moment. "Maybe... maybe I could touch his hand while Mama holds him?"

And that's what we did. Her finger traced his tiny palm while her mother held him close enough for Maria to smell his baby scent. The heart monitor showed what we could all feel—her rhythm settling as she touched her son.

"See?" I said softly. "Your heart knows him."

By the end of my shift, I realized I'd spent more time coaching people through their fears than I had adjusting IV drips. The conversations that mattered most weren't about medications or procedures—they were about the emotional scaffolding that holds people together when their bodies fall apart.

Walking to my car, I thought about Mr. Davidson learning to live with fear instead of being paralyzed by it, about Maria touching her baby's hand as her first step toward trust, about the man in Room 18 from yesterday, who finally identified the difference between strength and stubbornness.

These weren't accidents. They were appointments.

I pulled the TECU note from my pocket—the one I'd been

carrying since that dinner table conversation. The edges were soft now, worn from handling.

The Emotional Check-Up.

Maybe it was time to stop carrying it and start building it.

Later that evening, Virgil found me sitting on the curb outside, shoes off, hair wild, staring at the dark sky.

"You good?" he asked, plopping down beside me.

I shrugged. "Patients got me rethinking my whole life."

Virgil grinned. "Girl, join the club. We should get jackets."

I laughed, but it didn't shake the thought: maybe all these conversations—these accidental coaching moments— weren't accidents at all. Perhaps they were breadcrumbs.

**Coach T Says:** *Sometimes the conversations that stop us mid-chaos are the ones that shape us most. Listen closely. Your next chapter may already be whispering through someone else's story.*

# CHAPTER 14

# CHILI, CHAOS, AND CLARITY

Hospitals run on bad timing, and by 9:00 a.m., bad timing was serving us a three-course meal: three ambulance stretchers rolled in like a NASCAR pit crew, two visitors were screaming in stereo loud enough to rattle the vending machines, and somewhere down the hall, a Code Brown brewed in the air vents like it was Taco Tuesday.

The phones rang, the overhead paged, and the smell of burnt coffee mixed with Lysol told me it was going to be a long one.

Mai had barely clocked in when she poked her head into my bay, ponytail already listing to the side like it knew better. "Norma, today's gonna be messy."

I tugged on my gloves with a snap. "Messy is my baseline. Give me something new."

She didn't smile. Just raised one eyebrow. "No. I mean messy-messy. Mr. Lopez is back." She lowered her voice like she was delivering a horror movie twist. "Mask Rebel." I groaned. "Not the patron saint of dangling PPE."

Mr. Lopez—seventy-two years old, stubborn as a toddler at bedtime, lungs strong enough to inflate Macy's parade balloons—was perched in his bed like a king holding court. His surgical mask dangled from one ear like it had fainted halfway through its shift.

"Mr. Lopez," I said, planting my hands on my hips. "Why is your mask crying for help?"

He smirked. "Can't breathe with it on."

Mai folded her arms, eyebrow twitching so hard it looked ready to clock out. "You can breathe just fine. You don't like it."

He leaned back, eyes twinkling. "Feels like government control. Next thing you know, y'all gonna put GPS trackers in our IV bags."

"Sir," I said flatly, "the only thing in your IV bag is Lasix, and trust me—you'll know it's working in about ten minutes."

That shut him up for half a beat. He tugged the mask up, then let it slide down again like a toddler testing boundaries.

From the next bed over, a woman with a fractured ankle piped up. "I'll take the GPS if it means y'all can find my nurse faster."

Before I could respond, Nurse Carter strolled by, coffee in hand, and said matter-of-factly, "Ma'am, we tried that program last year. The nurses hid in radiology until it failed." Then he kept walking, as if it were just another Tuesday.

Mr. Lopez snorted so hard his mask popped back into place. "Fine. Arctic Tundra it is," he muttered.

Mai smirked as we walked out. "You're the only person I know who can win a mask standoff with sarcasm and a backup choir."

I sighed, tugging at my badge lanyard. One patient down, two screaming visitors, three stretchers, and God knows how many hours to go.

Norma: 1. Mask Rebel: 0. Burnout: still keeping score.

The overhead speaker blared: "Code spill—main hallway." Hospital translation: everybody grab a mop and pray.

When we arrived, I froze. A visitor had tripped over a flipflop, sending a cafeteria tray of chili flying like fireworks.

The hallway was now a river of beans and regret, slicking its way toward the electrical outlets.

A half-dozen medical students stood frozen in a huddle, clipboards out, whispering like David Attenborough narrating a wildlife scene. "Observe the wild nurse in her natural habitat," one muttered. "Should we... help?" another asked. "No," said the tallest, scribbling furiously. "This is enrichment. We're just here to observe."

A janitor leaned against his mop, shook his head, and muttered, "They don't pay me enough to clean Jackson

Pollock's chili period."

"Do you want mop or crowd control?" Mai asked.

I eyed the chili creeping closer to the outlets. "I'll take mop. You handle the baby doctors before they write a thesis on chili viscosity."

I was halfway through corralling the mess when a voice rang out from the waiting room. "Somebody get me a bowl and a spoon! Waste not, want not!"

Gasps followed. Then: "Ohhh, she's gonna fall!"

I spun just in time to see Mrs. Whitmore—church hat, orthopedic shoes, handbag lifted like Noah's Ark—tiptoeing across the slick floor like Moses testing the Red Sea.

"Mrs. Whitmore! Don't you dare—" Too late.

Her shoe hit chili. Arms windmilled like Looney Tunes. For one horrifying second, I saw the headline: 'Church Lady

Downed by Chili at County Hospital.'

Mai darted in, catching her just in time.

Mrs. Whitmore clutched her pearls. "Thank you, sugar. I'd hate to explain that to my bridge club."

From behind us, a visitor holding a Subway bag said,

"Honestly, smells better than what I ordered."

By the time housekeeping arrived, the hall looked like abstract art in shades of regret. One doctor peeked in, sniffed, and muttered, "Another day in paradise," before backing right out.

I stared at the mop in my hand, chili still creeping toward my shoes, and muttered, "If one more thing slides across this floor, it might be me."

I thought we were in the clear until Virgil called from the next bay. "Norma, you'd better come see this!"

Inside sat a young woman with abdominal pain and a morphine buzz. She was belting Whitney Houston's "I Will Always Love You" into her IV pole like it was a microphone. Every time we tried to assess her pain, she modulated higher.

"Ma'am," I said gently, "we need you to save some oxygen for breathing."

She pointed at me mid-note: "DON'T. YOU. TELL. ME. HOW. TO. LOVE."

I turned to Virgil. "You're on vocals tonight. I'm clocking out of this number."

As she hit the high note, three alarms beeped down the hall. My soul said: burnout incoming.

By mid-shift, I was running on caffeine, sarcasm, and pure adrenaline. My feet throbbed, my back ached, and my brain kept asking the same question: Is this it? Is this the rest of my life?

I ducked into the supply closet, leaned against a shelf of IV tubing, and let out a long breath. For a second, I wanted to stay there forever. Quiet. Still. No chili. No codes. No Whitney impersonators.

But the pager buzzed, reality snapped back, and I pushed off the wall.

By the time I stumbled into my house that night, the caffeine was gone, the spite had evaporated, and my bones were lobbying for early retirement.

The door swung open and greeted me with two things: burnt popcorn smoke curling through the air like a bad omen, and Kody barking like somebody owed him rent money.

"Kody!" I yelled.

My one-legged rescue came hopping proudly down the hall, tail wagging so hard it threatened to knock him over, my wig clamped between his teeth like a prize he'd won at the county fair.

Behind him, Ryan—my oldest—stood frozen in the kitchen doorway, clutching a mixing bowl like it was evidence.

"Mom, we tried to make snacks for movie night, but the microwave started smoking and—"

Dylan, my youngest, popped his head out from behind the couch, eyes wide with the kind of guilt only kids can carry. "—and then Kody attacked your mannequin head because we put sunglasses on it. He thought it was alive."

I blinked. Once. Twice. "So let me get this straight: the dog ate my hair, the popcorn tried to burn down the house, and my wig has officially retired. Anything else I should know?"

Dylan shrugged with Olympic-level nonchalance. "We also played bingo with your quarters. Ryan lost fifty cents."

Ryan shot him a look. "Because you called five numbers at once!"

I opened my mouth to lecture, but the sight of Kody prancing in circles with my wig—tilted just so, like RuPaul's onelegged cousin on a victory lap—undid me.

I laughed. Loud. Ugly. The kind of laugh that makes your stomach hurt, the kind you don't see coming but saves you from collapsing under the weight of everything else.

Later, after the smoke cleared and Kody finally surrendered the wig, curling up at my feet like nothing had happened, the boys surprised me.

No more jokes. No more chaos. Just stillness in the living room, the glow of the TV bouncing across their faces.

Ryan cleared his throat first, fiddling with the edge of his bowl. "Mom... I'm drowning in these college applications.

Everyone makes it sound easy, but it feels like my whole future is one big essay prompt."

Dylan leaned against me, his voice smaller than usual. "And I hate seeing you so tired all the time. Like... you're here, but you're not really here."

Their honesty cracked something open in me. It was the exact moment I've had with patients—the one where the noise fades, the beeping monitors blur, and the truth steps out into the open.

I swallowed, choosing my words carefully. "Y'all know

I'm not gonna be in this hospital forever, right?"

Ryan frowned. "Wait... are you retiring?"

I shook my head, smiling at the thought. "Not yet. But maybe... I'm figuring out another way to help people. A way that doesn't eat me alive before I make it home to you."

They didn't press. They didn't need to. The way they looked at me—half worried, half relieved—told me they understood more than I wanted to admit.

Later, when they'd gone to bed and the house was finally quiet, I sat on the edge of my own bed, staring at my scrubs folded neatly for the next day.

And that whisper inside me got louder.

Maybe my real work isn't in the hospital anymore. Perhaps it's in the space after. The space where I can breathe, and they can see me breathe, too.

**Coach T Says:** *Sometimes the chaos isn't there to drive you crazy—it's there to clear enough noise for you to hear yourself finally.*

# CHAPTER 15

# ONE FOOT OUT THE DOOR

The day started suspiciously calm. Which, if you've worked in a hospital for more than fifteen seconds, you know is the universe warming up its throwing arm.

The board looked blessedly manageable. No one was yelling. No alarms were tail-spinning. The air even smelled less like bleach and more like coffee and floor wax, which I took personally.

"Don't say it," Denise warned, passing me in the hall with a stack of charts. "Don't you even whisper the Q-word." "I wasn't," I lied. "I was gonna say... it's very—"

Her face went horror-movie still. "Absolutely not."

"Fine." I sipped my coffee so dark it could file a complaint.

"I won't say it's... quiet."

Three beats.

A bed alarm screamed like a tornado siren. Somewhere behind me, a voice yelled, "I'm escaping!" And, as if choreographed, a rolling linen cart banged into a doorjamb and sneezed towels like confetti.

"Now look," Denise huffed. "You spoke it into existence."

"I'm a prophet," I said, jogging toward the noise. "Pay me in hazard pay and sweet tea."

Room 9's door was half open, and there he was: Mr. Ned, late seventies, wearing white socks and a gown tied around his waist like a makeshift belt, apparently because it was superhero day, with an ankle bracelet monitor blinking "absolutely not." He was halfway into one of those hospital wheelchairs that require an engineering degree to operate. It was facing the wrong direction. He straddled it like a horse nobody asked for.

"Sir," I said, putting on my polite voice. "Where are we

going in such a hurry?"

"I have to feed the meter," he announced. "They'll tow me."

"Sir, you arrived by ambulance."

Pause. His eyes skittered left. "Then I have to feed... the fish."

"You don't have fish."

He considered this. "I might."

I eased the chair back and helped him sit. "Let's feed the fish in a few hours. After your chest X-ray, deal?"

He nodded. "Fine. But I'm stealing Jell-O."

"Make it lemon so housekeeping can't tell on you," I whispered, steering him back to bed. He grinned like we were co-conspirators. I tucked him in, smoothed the blanket, and set his call bell where he could find it with his eyes closed.

Back at the nurses' station, Mai was engaged in delicate diplomacy with a woman carrying two overflowing "Get Well" gift bags.

"If the Jell-O leaves the room, ma'am, it stops being Jell-O and starts being theft," Mai said kindly.

The woman clutched her pearls. "But it's for my sister. For comfort."

"We also offer comfort in the form of blankets and nurses with good cheekbones," I chimed in. "Return the Jell-O; keep your dignity."

She surrendered a six-pack like we'd cornered her in a parking garage. "You two are very mean," she told us.

"We prefer efficient," Mai said, stacking the cups like trophies.

"Also," I added, "healthcare markup on contraband Jell-O would bankrupt you."

We were still smirking when the unit phone rang. The kind of ring that says: someone important wants something you don't have time to give. I scooped it up.

"ED nurses' station, this is Norma."

A bright, too-cheerful voice answered. "Hi! I'm Lila with Community Partners Network. We're piloting a free emotional wellness series for frontline families and are seeking a lead facilitator. Your name came up. Twice."

"Twice?" I echoed, side-eyeing the ceiling like there was a camera up there. "Who did this to me?"

She chuckled. "A respiratory therapist named Joy and a charge nurse named Rivera. They said you have a way with people."

I blew air out of my cheeks. "Debatable. What is it, exactly?"

"Two-hour workshop in two weeks. Saturday morning.

Community center on Orchard. The topic is Grounding in Chaos. We pay a modest honorarium—and we cover materials."

My brain flicked through excuses like a Rolodex on fastforward. I don't have time. I don't do microphones. I smell like chlorhexidine most days. And yet.

Grounding in Chaos.

"Lila," I said slowly, "you realize I work the world's most unpredictable schedule."

"Totally," she chirped. "I can send a sample outline. You tweak it. We'll handle the rest."

I pinched my nose. "Let me call you back by the end of the day?"

"Perfect. I'll email you now."

I hung up. Mai stared. "Who was that?"

"Fate," I said, trying to keep my face casual and failing. "Or spam. Hard to say."

Before she could press, an overhead voice bellowed, "Security to triage." The pitch of the unit changed, a subtle hush before the crowd leans in. Denise's eyebrows made a high arc. "Five says it's Carl."

"I'll take that action," I said, and we hustled.

Triage was a scene. Security Rogers had his hands on his hips, doing his "I am tired of this" stance. A teenager recorded on her phone while her father pretended not to notice. The volunteer at the desk was fanning herself with patient stickers.

And in the middle of it all—of course—stood a well-known, heavily perfumed visitor with a tote bag stuffed suspiciously full, arguing about why she was allowed to "take a few extra pudding cups because they were unopened."

Carl? Not visible. But the tote bag rustled.

"Do not," I whispered to the universe. "Do not."

The tote shimmied like a live thing. A small paw emerged, patted the air once, and disappeared.

"Oh for the love of tiny bandits," I muttered. "Ma'am, is there a raccoon in your bag?"

She clutched it closer. "It's a cat."

"That is a lie told by someone who has never met a cat," I said, reaching for the strap. Rogers stepped in, surprisingly gentle, and the bag released a resigned little chirp.

Carl, eyes bright and shameless, peered out like, What? I brought my own container.

"Ma'am," Rogers said, voice silked with exasperation, "you cannot smuggle wildlife through triage."

She sniffed. "He likes Jell-O."

"We all like Jell-O," I said. "That's not the bar."

While Rogers performed a raccoon eviction with the patience of a Methodist, I guided the queue forward, because the secret of triage is you keep the river moving no matter who swims through it.

By the time housekeeping came to wipe down the sink, Carl was escorted toward the loading dock like a celebrity being led to a limo after embarrassing himself in public. Again.

Back at the station, Mai touched my elbow. "You okay?"

I realized my heart was doing that drumline thing.

Adrenaline had a signature. I knew it too well.

"Yeah," I said. "Just thinking about a thing."

"A good thing?"

"A maybe thing."

She nodded, as if that made all the sense in the world.

We rolled into midday. A teenager with panic attacks who didn't want her mother to know. An older woman with a bruise shaped like silence. A man insisting he was fine while his skin told a different story. I toggled between stingy and soft, between fast and present. The dance I know.

During a rare lull, I opened the email from Lila. The subject line was bright—Workshop Outline: Grounding in

Chaos— and the attachment read like she'd seen inside my head:

Opening circle. Naming the storm. Breath that doesn't feel corny. "One-minute resets" you can do in a bathroom stall at work. Boundaries that don't start fights. Closing ritual with pockets full of hope.

My palms went warm.

Virgil plopped into the chair across from me, tray clattering.

"You look like you're about to quit mid-bite," he said.

I smiled. "Not quitting. Just... questioning."

He studied me. "Norma, if you ever leave this place, it'll fall apart. Who else is gonna wrangle Mask Rebel and chili spills?"

"Somebody will," I said. "But maybe I'm supposed to be doing more than just wrangling. Maybe I'm supposed to be helping people untangle what the medicine can't touch."

He raised an eyebrow. "Like a therapist?"

I shook my head slowly. "Not exactly. More like... a coach. For the messy parts, nobody charts."

Virgil let out a low whistle. "Coach Norma. Has a ring to it."

I laughed, but my chest felt lighter, like he'd named something I hadn't dared say out loud.

The afternoon clattered into evening the way it always does—gurneys, clipboards, someone crying, someone laughing too loud because they survived a thing they didn't think they would. I wrote the discharge instructions that double as lullabies. I charted like a poet on a deadline. I forgot to eat the half-banana I'd tucked in my pocket until it had thoughts and a philosophy degree.

By clock-out, my feet ached in that good, punished way. The kind of ache that says, You earned your shower. I called Lila from the parking lot, watching dusk flatten the edges of the building.

"Okay," I said when she picked up. "I'll do it."

Her relief was audible. "Yes! You won't regret it. I'll send you logistics."

"Please do. And... Lila?"

"Yeah?"

"Keep the 'lead facilitator' part quiet. My job is... my job." "Understood," she said, and I believed her.

At home, the house smelled like laundry detergent and boys. Ryan was sprawled on the couch with a textbook open, but had read zero pages. Dylan had a mixing bowl and a face dusted with flour, like a toddler who had lost a fight with a donut. Kody hopped over, barked once, and face-planted into my shins, which is his love language.

"Family meeting," I announced, grabbing two mismatched mugs and filling them with tap water because self-care is sometimes just hydration.

Both heads turned. The TV clicked off. We gathered at the kitchen table—the epicenter of our lives, the surface where bills, bingo cards, and miracles get sorted.

"I said yes to a workshop," I told them. "Two Saturdays from now. Emotional wellness stuff. Just... me doing the thing I keep doing in hallways."

Ryan's eyebrows climbed. "Like... coaching?"

"Like... not therapy," I said. "But not coaching."

Dylan grinned. "You gonna be TikTok famous?"
"Absolutely not," I said, and the lie tasted almost sweet. "But I might make someone's day better."

Ryan considered me, older than he is, for one second.

"Sounds like you're finally doing something for you."

Sometimes your children sneak up on you and hold up a mirror without even meaning to. "Maybe I am," I admitted.

Two weeks later, on a Saturday morning that began so blue it hurt, I parked outside the Orchard Community Center. The building wasn't special—just concrete block and civic pride—but there were flowers planted by a Girl Scout troop, leaning bravely against the stairs. Inside, someone had made coffee and arranged folding chairs in a circle, as if they believed in the possibility of something happening between strangers.

"Norma!" Lila waved, cheeks as earnest as her emails. "You look perfect."

"I look like I ironed my scrubs," I said. "Which I did not."

We laid out clipboards, pens, and a small bowl of Jolly Ranchers, because sugar serves as moral support. People trickled in: a bus driver, a kindergarten teacher, a mom with three kids in tow, a security guard I recognized from nights, and—my breath caught—a respiratory therapist from our hospital who'd only ever nodded at me in passing. She sat, eyes down, fingers brittle around a paper cup.

I started like I start with patients who don't want to be here.

"Hi. I'm Norma. I wash my hands when I'm nervous, and I fuss when I care. I don't have your answers. I do have some tools, and if they don't fit, you can discard them. No hard feelings."

We talked. Lord, we spoke about panic pretending to be anger. About taking five breaths in a bathroom stall because it's the only door you can lock. About the mean voice in your head, you'd never let near a child. About what you can say to someone who is falling apart that doesn't require a cape or a counseling degree.

I taught a one-minute reset that doesn't feel silly if you do it with both feet heavy and hands on your own shoulders, as if you're not a visitor in your own body. People practiced. People cried. People laughed because crying felt like admitting something important.

We closed with the index cards. "Write down a sentence you want to hear next time it's too much," I said. "Write it like it's from someone who loves you with their whole chest." They wrote: 'You're allowed to rest.' 'You don't have to fix it today.' 'You still get to be a person.'

The security guard approached me after, card in hand. "I'm gonna put this in my wallet," he said, throat thick. "Next to my badge."

"Good," I said, and the word felt bigger than it is.

We stacked chairs. We wiped tables. Lila hugged me like she was holding onto a co-conspirator. My phone buzzed with three new messages: one from a person asking for resources, another from a nurse on another unit inquiring if I'd consider attending their staff meeting, and a cousin sending me a meme about bingo night.

In the parking lot, the day was warm enough to soften the edges. I sat in my car and let silence sit in the front seat like an honored guest. Something in me that had been clenched for years uncurled an inch.

Then my pager—yes, my dinosaur, faithful, chain-on-thehip- hip pager—vibrated against my waistband, rattling the quiet like a cup on a Jurassic Park dashboard.

ED CALLBACK -- STAT.

I stared at the number. It blinked like a heartbeat. I could feel the hospital pulling like a tide. It always will.

I looked back at the community center, still smelling faintly of coffee and Jolly Ranchers and whatever it is that happens when people tell the truth near each other. Then down at the workshop outline in my lap, edges dog-eared, notes scrawled, a doodle of Kody wearing a little crown because why not.

I breathed. In. Out. Counted to five because I tell other people to do that, and I'm not a hypocrite. I pressed call.

"This is Norma," I said. "I'm on my way."

I tucked the index cards into my bag—the extras, blank and waiting—and drove toward the sirens, toward the place that made me, toward the next scene in a story I hadn't finished writing, not by a long shot.

One foot out the door. One foot is still inside. Both of them mine.

**Coach T says, *"The storm doesn't last forever."*** *There's always a pause, a quiet, a moment where the path shows itself. When it does—don't just notice it. Step into it.*

# COMING SOON

**Nurse Norma Chronicles: From Africa with Love, Lies, and Lessons**

A Journey of Passion, Heartbreak, and the Power to Begin Again.

She thought Africa would be her escape from call bells, chaos, and a loveless life. Instead, it became the place where passion, heartbreak, and hard truths collided.

In Nurse Norma Chronicles: From Africa with Love, Lies, and Lessons, Norma Jean Woods finally takes a breath away from the hospital halls and dives headfirst into her own story. From the breathtaking romance of a hot, steamy romance with a charming prince to the shocking unraveling of a marriage torn by tradition, Norma learns that love alone isn't enough when your power and peace are on the line.

This isn't just a love story. It's a story of rediscovery, resilience, and the courage it takes to say goodbye in order to begin again. Funny, raw, heartbreaking, and deeply relatable—Norma's African journey will leave every woman who's ever loved and lost nodding, laughing, and crying along with her.

150 Passion. Pain. Power.

Norma's transformation into Coach T gets juicier and richer with every new book—so stay on the ride, because her story is only getting started.

Get ready for Norma's most unforgettable chapter yet.

150

www.ingramcontent.com/pod-product-compliance
Lightning Source LLC
LaVergne TN
LVHW050913210926
848482LV00012B/427